Crisis:
Prevention and Response in the Community

Crisis:
Prevention and Response in the Community

Edited by
Ronald H. Hanson, PhD
Norman A. Wieseler, PhD
K. Charlie Lakin, PhD

David L. Braddock, PhD
AAMR Books and Research
Monographs Editor

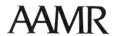

American Association on Mental Retardation

Published by
American Association on Mental Retardation
444 North Capitol Street, N.W., Suite 846
Washington, DC 20001-1512

Library of Congress Cataloging-in-Publication Data

Crisis: Prevention and response in the community / edited by Ronald H. Hanson, Norman A. Wieseler, K. Charlie Lakin.

    p. cm.
Includes bibliographical references.
ISBN 0-940898-74-8 (pbk.)
    1. Crisis intervention (Mental health services).   2. Community health services.
3. Counseling.   I. Hanson, Ronald Halton.   II. Wieseler, Norman Anthony.
III. Lakin, K. Charlie.

RC480.6 . C7585 2002
363.2'2--dc21   2002018379

Contributors

Richard W. Albin, PhD
University of Oregon
Eugene, Oregon

Daniel Baker, PhD
Oregon Rehabilitation Association
Salem, Oregon

Anjali Barretto, MA
University of Iowa
Iowa City, Iowa

Joan B. Beasley, PhD
Consultation and Training Services
Brookline, Massachusetts

Wendy K. Berg, MA
University of Iowa
Iowa City, Iowa

Jody S. Britten, MSEd
University of Kansas
Lawrence, Kansas

Karen Craven, BA
Oregon Rehabilitation Association
Salem, Oregon

Patrick Frawley, PhD
Vermont Crisis Intervention Network
Moretown, Vermont

Rachel Freeman, PhD
University of Kansas
Lawrence, Kansas

Ronald H. Hanson, PhD, FAAMR
Mount Olivet Rolling Acres
Victoria, Minnesota

Jay Harding, EdS
University of Iowa
Iowa City, Iowa

Peter Holmes, PhD
Eastern Michigan University
Ypsilanti, Michigan

Robert Horner, PhD
University of Oregon
Eugene, Oregon

Jeri Kroll, MDiv
Greater Lynn Mental Health and
    Retardation Center
Lynn, Massachusetts

K. Charlie Lakin, PhD
University of Minnesota
Minneapolis, Minnesota

Sheryl A. Larson, PhD
University of Minnesota
Minneapolis, Minnesota

Amy McCart, MSEd
University of Kansas
Shawnee, Kansas

Joan M. Oslund, MA
Mount Olivet Rolling Acres
Victoria, Minnesota

Christopher L. Smith, PhD
University of Kansas
Lawrence, Kansas

Michael W. Smull, BA
Support Development Association
Annapolis, Maryland

Lamar Trant, PsyD
Colorado Bluesky Enterprises, Inc.
Pueblo, Colorado

Elia Vecchione, PhD
Vermont Crisis Intervention Network
Moretown, Vermont

Lawrence A. Velasco, MEd
Colorado Bluesky Enterprises, Inc.
Pueblo, Colorado

David P. Wacker, PhD
University of Iowa
Iowa City, Iowa

Gregory A. Wagner, PhD
California Department of Developmental
    Services
Sacramento, California

Norman A. Wieseler, PhD
Eastern Minnesota Community Support
    Services
Faribault, Minnesota

Steven G. Zelenski, DO, PhD
Central Wisconsin Center for the
    Developmentally Disabled
Madison, Wisconsin

Table of Contents

List of Tables

List of Figures

INTRODUCTION

Reflecting on the 20th century, we note the deinstitutionalization movement as the most prominent influence in enriching the lives of people with intellectual disabilities. The change from large congregate care facilities to more integrated community-based settings has required profound alterations in the design and provision of services.

Crisis services — the prevention and minimization of dangerous and destructive behaviors and the organized effective response when the crisis situation occurs — has emerged nationwide as a necessary service. Organized, systematic crisis prevention and response can minimize inappropriate and costly alternatives, such as emergency psychiatric hospitalizations, or restrictive, punitive reactions, such as incarcerations. As states or smaller regional collaborative partners provide good crisis services, they can help ensure the success of their deinstitutionalization efforts.

This publication provides important information to readers who are planning crisis services and describes how such services are currently being provided in many different states or locales. Part 1 examines the challenge of community systems. Part 2 addresses state and regional networks of crisis prevention and response. Part 3 presents specialized programs designed for special populations.

In chapter 1 Charlie Lakin and Sheryl Larson provide a summary of the past, present, and future of community residential, vocational, and other services for people with developmental disabilities. They describe what has been learned in the development of community-based services and examine the major challenges in sustaining and expanding community living opportunities, particularly as they relate to those individuals traditionally viewed as difficult to serve or unlikely to adjust to community living. In the next chapter, Ronald Hanson and Norman Wieseler identify the many forces that influenced the development and provision of crisis services in Minnesota. These authors review the characteristics and needs of people who have used crisis prevention and response services. They address issues in systems planning and the consultative role in the provision of crisis services.

Part 2 describes state and regional networks of behavioral support and crisis services. In chapter 3 Patrick Frawley and Elia Vecchione describe the Vermont Crisis Intervention Network, a collaborative program between the regional mental health centers and the state division of mental retardation. Chapter 4 by Norman Wieseler, Ronald Hanson, and Joan Oslund presents Minnesota's public-private collaboration in providing crisis services. The way in which they conjointly address crisis needs of individual clients in the Twin Cities metro area is described. In chapter 5 Gregory Wagner discusses the behavioral and crisis services available in California. He reviews the California system of regional responsibility and the history of the class action lawsuit that increased the rate of deinstitutionalization. The final chapter in this part describes the START/Sovner Center Program in Massachusetts. Authors Joan Beasley and Jeri Kroll present the program's history, philosophy, service elements, and current status. They also share evaluation results.

Part 3 presents specialized programs for special populations. In chapter 7 David Wacker, Jay Harding, Wendy Berg, and Anjali Barretto describe the outreach services from the University of Iowa Clinic, discussing the model, funding, and challenges to sustained support. A summary is also provided of follow-up data on the participants served. Lawrence Velasco, Lamar Trant, and Peter Holmes discuss in chapter 8 the Colorado multisystem collaborative process in diversion or creative sentencing to prevent hospitalization and incarceration. The focus is upon the Pueblo Developmental Disabilities/Mental Health Consortium. The members work together to provide treatment and other ongoing community support. This is followed by a discussion of training, technical assistance, and consultation for support staff to prevent and respond to behavioral crises. Authors Daniel Baker, Richard Albin, Karen Craven, and Norman Wieseler in chapter 9 give special emphasis to the inclusion of all members of the interdisciplinary team and positive incident-based planning for behavioral support. Chapter 10 describes functional and systems-level assessment. Authors Rachel Freeman, Daniel Baker, Robert Horner, Chris Smith, Jody Britten, and Amy McCart describe a systems approach in providing behavioral support to clients in need of crisis services. Chapter 11 by Michael Smull describes the philosophy and practice of person-centered planning and its application in North Carolina as an intervention for challenging and crisis-causing behavior. In chapter 12 Steven Zelenski discusses and evaluates the use of psychopharmacologic treatment as part of crisis intervention, providing a thorough and comprehensive discussion on the treatment of mental health emergencies. The final chapter, by Norman Wieseler and Ronald Hanson, discusses team planning and team building for preventing and responding to individual crises. It details the integration of disciplines and how each contributes to the overall individualized service plan.

Ronald H. Hanson
Norman A. Wieseler
July 2002

PART 1

The Challenge of Community Systems

CHAPTER 1

The Social and Policy Context of Community-Centered Behavioral Supports and Crisis Response

K. Charlie Lakin
Sheryl A. Larson
University of Minnesota
Minneapolis, Minnesota

The Social Movement Toward Community Living for All

Over the last three decades of the 20th century, the United States witnessed remarkable achievements in reducing the populations of people with mental retardation and related developmental disabilities (MR-DD) in public institutions. Between June 1967 and June 2000, the number of people with MR-DD residing in both state MR-DD and psychiatric institutions was reduced by 79%, from 228,500 to 48,080 (Prouty & Lakin, 2001). Populations of state MR-DD institutions (16 or more residents) decreased by 76%, from 194,650 to 47,592 during this period. In June 2000 only 12.6% of people receiving MR-DD residential services outside their family homes lived in state institutions and only 22.0% lived in either public or private institutions of 16 or more residents (Prouty & Lakin, 2001). When deinstitutionalization was just beginning in 1969, the Master Facility Inventory of the United States showed only 10,350 people with MR-DD living in community residential settings of 15 or fewer residents (4% of the total of institution-and-community residents) (Lakin, Hill, & Bruininks, 1985); by 2000, 292,013 people with MR-DD lived in community settings (78% of all institution-and-community residents) (Prouty, Smith & Lakin, 2001).

The massive depopulation of state institutions and associated inefficiencies of operating them at far below their capacity have pushed the nationwide per resident average annual expenditure to more than $100,000 per year ($108,000 in fiscal year [FY] 1999; Prouty & Lakin, 2000). The experience of successfully providing community services to people who in the past would have been institutionalized has also increased the skill, experience, and confidence in a growing number of states to conclude that institutions are an unnecessary component of state service systems. As a result of state commitments to provide community services to all who can benefit and to eliminate unjustifiably costly services, in the 12 years between 1988 and 1999, 116 state MR-DD institutions and MR-DD units of 16 or more residents within traditional psychiatric institutions were closed. This represented more than one third (33.6%) of all state MR-DD institutions and units that have operated since 1960. Including the 33 state institution closures before 1988, by 1999 only 56% of all state institutions operating in or established after 1960 remained in operation. Ten states have effectively closed all state MR-DD institutions.

The most visible product of the deinstitutionalization movement in the United States has been the depopulation of institutions, but the most important accomplishment has been the concurrent transfer of the full range of services once available only in institutions to the communities in which people are born and in which they prefer to live. Today the vast majority of service recipients and over two thirds (72%) of service expenditures are in the community (Braddock, Hemp, Parish, & Rizzolo, 2000). Most people with MR-DD who receive services today do so without ever having experienced a day of institutionalization. Indeed, it is statistically demonstrable that the primary factor in the massive depopulation of state institutions has not been the number of people discharged from state institutions but the reduction in the number of people who entered state institutions. To exemplify, between 1970 and 1998, annual admissions to state MR-DD institutions decreased 84% while discharges decreased 68% (Prouty & Lakin, 1999).

One trend that has notably distinguished the deinstitutionalization movement for people with MR-DD has been that as institutional services have been reduced, commensurate amounts of services and resources have been developed in the community. To exemplify, in 1999 the reported numbers of people with MR-DD receiving institutional and community (out-of-family home) residential services per 100,000 of the general population was 132.4, a rate that was little changed from the ratio of 130.4 in 1967 (Prouty & Lakin, 2000). Of course with national population growth, the total number of residential service recipients in MR-DD systems also grew (from 230,000 in 1967 to 361,172 in 1999).

Another important feature of this same movement, with its focus on community support and culturally typical experiences, has been the dramatic reduction in the number of children and youth (0 to 21 years) living in state institutions (from 91,592 in 1965 to 2,471 in 1998). Equally important is the reduction in the number of children and youth with MR-DD in all forms of out-of-home residential settings (from 91,000 in June 1977 to 24,000 in June 1997) (Lakin, Anderson, & Prouty, 1998). Such statistics reflect a growing commitment and capability of communities throughout the United States to accommodate people with a wide range of support needs, including people whose extensive support needs would have assured them admission to institutional settings in years past.

The Compelling Outcomes of Community Living

The pace of deinstitutionalization and the movement of people and services for them into the community would have been unsustainable if the people affected had not experienced positive outcomes. Documentation of positive outcomes of community living continues to stimulate state efforts to make available community living opportunities and needed supports to groups of individuals once considered appropriately institutionalized, including people with behavioral and emotional disabilities. The substantial body of research and evaluation focused on the outcomes of community services for people with MR-DD in areas such as (a) functional skills development, (b) social relationships, (c) community participation, and (d) family satisfaction.

Functional Skills

In 1989 and 1999 exhaustive reviews were conducted of research and evaluation studies focused on the functional skills ("adaptive behavior" or basic daily living skills) associated with moving from institutional to community settings (Kim, Larson, & Lakin, 2001; Larson & Lakin, 1989). In all, 27 deinstitutionalization studies were published in the United States between 1980 and 1999 that met the following criteria: (a) a minimum of five people moving from an institution to the community, (b) basic demographic and diagnostic information on the subjects, (c) primarily adult subjects, (d) baseline data collected prior to or within one month of moving to community, (e) postmovement data collected 6 months or longer from date of move, and (f) comprehensive adaptive behavior skills data collected at baseline and after move with the same adaptive behavior instrument. These studies included both: (a) contrast group studies in which outcomes for people moving were compared with a statistically equivalent group remaining behind and (b) longitudinal studies in which functional skills were assessed for the same group of individuals as they moved from institutions to the community.

Contrast Group Studies

Nine studies reported between 1980 and 1999 compared overall functional skills or adaptive behavior of people who moved from institutions to community residential settings (Bradley, Conroy, Covert, & Feinstein, 1986; Calapai, 1988; Conroy, Efthimiou, & Lemanowicz, 1982; Conroy, Lemanowicz, Feinstein, & Bernotsky, 1991; D'Amico, Hannah, Milhouse, & Froleich, 1978; Davis, 1990; Rosen, 1985; Schroeder & Hanes, 1978; Williams, Paskow, Thompson, & Levine, 1985). These studies varied from 12 to 72 months between baseline (institution) and follow-up assessments. Their number of subjects ranged from 13 to 248 individuals. In all nine of the studies, the direction of outcomes favored the group of people who moved out of the institutions, although in only six studies did the magnitude of change reach statistical significance (p < .05). Four other studies examined specific areas of adaptive behavior, but not overall adaptive behavior (Close, 1977; Eastwood & Fisher, 1988; Fuess, 1987; Horner, Stoner, & Ferguson, 1988). Areas examined included academic skills, community living skills, communication skills, physical skills, self-care and domestic skills, social skills, and vocational skills. The groups studied ranged from 12 to 122 subjects and the follow-up periods ranged from 12 to 50 months. In these studies a total of 17 separate comparisons were made within six areas of adaptive behavior. Better outcomes were obtained by movers in 15 comparisons, 9 of which reached statistical significance. In two areas no numerical differences were obtained.

Longitudinal Studies
A total of 18 studies were conducted between 1980 and 1999 to examine changes in the adaptive behavior of a single group of people who left institutions to live in community settings (Apgar, Cook, & Lerman, 1998; Bolin, 1994; Bradley et al., 1986; Calapai, 1988; Center for Outcome Analysis, 1999; Colorado Division of Developmental Disabilities, 1982; Conroy & Bradley, 1985; Conroy, Feinstein, & Lemanowicz, 1988; Conroy et al., 1991; Conroy, Seiders, & Yuskauskus, 1998; Conroy, 1995, 1998; Fortune, Heinlein, & Fortune, 1995; Rose, White, Conroy, & Smith, 1993; Thompson & Carey, 1980; Williams et al., 1985). These groups ranged in size from 7 to 569 people. Sample members were followed from 6 to 72 months. Sixteen of the 18 studies found numerically higher adaptive behavior among sample members after they moved to the community, with differences reaching statistical significance in 13 of the studies. In three studies numerical improvements in adaptive behavior scores did not reach statistical significance. In one study people moving to the community experienced statistically significant decrease in adaptive behavior. In one other study subjects experienced a statistically significant decrease in adaptive behavior in their first 6 months in the community with subsequent statistically significant increases in the next 6-month and 18-month periods, but with no comparisons with the original baseline.

Such findings have provided high levels of support for the relative power of community services and experiences in supporting the development of functional skills among people with MR-DD. Because these studies have included people with a full range of intellectual disabilities, they supported the proposition that systems of services that are willing to provide all essential functions and "safety

nets" within the community can successfully operate as "all-community systems."
States and local governments and quasigovernmental administrative units are
making the commitment to do so, not only because people "develop" better in the
community, but because they live better in the community.

Social Relationships

Although research on the involvement of family members in the lives of people
with MR-DD has shown the difficulty of reestablishing family relationships (e.g.,
a majority of people moving to community settings from institutions do not
reestablish monthly or more frequent contact with family members), they do experience considerably more family contact in the community than they did while
an institution resident (Eastwood, 1985; Feinstein, Lemanowicz, & Conroy,
1988; Stancliffe & Lakin, 1998). Studies have also shown considerably more frequent family contact for residents in community settings who have not experienced prior institutionalization than for former institutional residents, but such
comparisons are confounded by age and severity of disability (Hill et al., 1989).

Direct comparisons of family involvement in the lives of people living in community group homes with relatively fewer versus relatively more residents have
also shown people living with fewer other residents to have more family involvement in their lives (Feinstein, Lemanowicz, Spreat, & Conroy, 1986; Hill et al.,
1989); that is, the number of people with whom one shares housing has an inverse
relationship with the number of times family members visit the house.

Willer and Intagliata (1980) also found that the social interactions of people
in community residential settings was affected not only by the characteristics of
the residents, but also by the number of people in the home, controlling for resident
age and level of functioning.

The most powerful factor in the establishment of social relationships for people with as well as without disabilities is regular, ongoing social contact (Abery &
Fahnestock, 1994; Abery, Thurlow, Johnson, & Bruininks, 1990). More specifically, adults with MR-DD more predictably develop social relationships when
they have access to and participate in activities that are likely to result in social interaction and that frequently take place. Institutional life is consistently shown to
yield substantially smaller social networks than community settings (Conroy, Seiders, & Yuskauskis, 1998; Horner, Stoner, & Ferguson, 1988), presumably because institutional life is consistently shown to be inferior to community living in
providing access to community participation, which contributes directly to social
relationships.

Community Participation

The social and community participation of people living in community settings
is impressively and consistently greater than that of people living in institutions.
Numerous studies have shown outcomes favoring community life in areas in-

cluding: (a) frequency of going to movies, restaurants, sporting events, and other forms of public entertainment; (b) frequency of visiting stores to purchase clothing, food, and other items of necessity and choice; (c) frequency of going out, visiting friends, and using public transportation to go where people want; (d) frequency of participating in organized sports; (e) numbers of friendships with non-handicapped people; (f) frequency of going places with one's own family; and (g) frequency of attendance at community religious services and activities (Conroy, Seiders, & Yuskauskas, 1998; Conroy & Bradley, 1985; Conroy, 1998; Felce, de Kock, & Repp, 1986; Horner, Stoner, & Ferguson, 1988; O'Neill, Brown, Gordon, & Schonhorn, 1981; Stancliffe & Lakin, 1998).

Family Attitudes and Satisfaction

More than a dozen studies of parent attitudes and experiences with deinstitutionalization and community placement provide substantial support from families of the benefits of movement to the community for their family members. A 1991 review of 21 studies (Larson & Lakin, 1991) found that while the vast majority (about 80% on average) of family members of people in institutions were satisfied with their family members' institutions, parents viewed the institutions less favorably after the move and were overwhelmingly positive about community living. Subsequent research in California by Conroy, Seiders, and Yuskauskas (1998) has shown the same tendencies, with 85% of parents in a sample of California's Coffelt class saying they would not want their family members returned to the institutions even though only 42% reported initially being in favor of the move out of the institution. Studies of family satisfaction have offered many suggestions by families about how families engaged in providing important supports to people moving from institutional to community settings (Larson & Lakin, 1991). These include: (a) attending and responding to the perceptions, needs, and concerns of family members regarding program design and the adequacy of the amounts and types of support needed in various community settings; (b) facilitating participation of the individual and family in decision making about changes in the person's life (e.g., where, when, with whom); (c) arranging opportunities for family members to learn about and visit potential service providers and evaluate their approaches and skills with the needs of individuals; (d) providing real choices for consumers and families in selecting residential and vocational services and service providers; and (e) establishing and maintaining effective communication and promoting family participation between service providers and family members after placement. Most important, service systems must develop capacities to avoid initial institutional placements that drag families through unnecessary and unproductive periods of life and life change.

Community Placement and Behavioral/Psychiatric Outcomes

The powerful, well-researched association between movement from institutional settings to community living and the acquisition of functional skills has been a significant factor in the continued support of depopulation of institutions. The evidence is very strong to support community living being a powerful, albeit loosely defined, treatment model for adaptive behavior skill growth. Studies of the association between community placement and changes in maladaptive (or "challenging") behavior have also tended to favor community living over institutional living, but have shown much less evidence of statistically significant effects or highly consistent findings.

There were between 1980 and 1999 six studies that directly compared maladaptive behavior changes among people deinstitutionalized and matched groups of people remaining in institutions (Bradley et al., 1986; Conroy, Efthimiou, & Lemanowicz, 1982; Conroy et al., 1991; Davis, 1990; Williams et al., 1985; Molony & Taplin, 1990). These studies followed about 700 subjects over periods ranging from 12 to 72 months. In only one of the studies did any of the differences reach statistical significance (Conroy, Efthimiou, & Lemanowicz, 1982). That study indicated statistically significant relative improvements in maladaptive behavior among like people moving to the community. In two of the other studies, maladaptive behavior change favored those moving to the community; in two, those staying in the institution; in one, the results were not statistically significant and were not reported so as to show this tendency.

In addition to the contrast group studies, there were a total 18 longitudinal studies of overall maladaptive behavior of people leaving institutions with baseline assessments in the institutions and follow-up assessments after a minimum of 6 months (and a maximum of 84 months) in the community. These studies are summarized in Table 1.1.

Of the 18 studies, 5 showed significant, positive changes in the overall or specific aspects of maladaptive behavior of subjects who moved to the community (Conroy, 1995; Conroy, Seiders, & Yuskauskas, 1998; Feinstein et al., 1986; Fortune, Heinlein, & Fortune, 1995; Rose et al., 1993). Two studies showed statistically significant negative changes in maladaptive behavior after people moved to the community (Conroy, Feinstein, & Lemanowicz, 1988; Williams et al., 1985), although in the case of one, the significantly negative change over the institution baseline was still a statistically significantly better outcome than experienced by a contrast group that remained institutionalized. Of the remaining, eight studies showed nonsignificant improvement with the move to the community, and three showed nonsignificant worsening of maladaptive behavior in the community. One reported no difference without reporting actual raw data.

The more consistent association between adaptive behavior improvements

TABLE 1.1

Changes in Challenging Behavior Over Time Association With Movement From Institutions to Community Settings, U.S., 1980–1999

Study	Location	N	Level of MR	Duration	Overall maladaptive	Internal	External	Asocial	Frequency	Severity
Apgar, Cook, & Lerman (1998)	NJ	44	All	60	+		+			
Bolin (1994)	OK	44	All	12					+	+
Bradley et al. (1986)	NH	93	All	84	-					
Business Services Group (1999)	CA	44	All	12	+					
Center for Outcome Analysis (1999)	IN	92	All	6	-					
Conroy (1995)	OK	382	All	60						++
Conroy (1998)	KS	88	Profound	12	+					
Conroy & Bradley (1985)	PA	383	All	72	+					
Conroy, Feinstein, & Lemanowicz (1988)	CT	207	All	24	--					
Conroy et al. (1991)	CT	569	All	60	+					
Conroy, Seiders, & Yuskauskas (1998)	CA	91	All	36	++					
Feinstein et al. (1986)	LA	158	All	9	++					
Fortune, Heinlein, & Fortune	WY	157	All	72	++	++	+	++		
Hayden et al. (1995)	MN	190	All	12	-*					
Horner, Stoner, & Ferguson (1988)	OR	23	All	60			+	+		
Kleinberg & Galligan (1983)	NJ	20	All	12	-					
Rose et al. (1993)	PA	7	Mild, Moderate	12	+	++	+	0		
Williams et al. (1985)	DC	80	All	15	--	--	--			

Note: ++ = statistically significant positive change; – – = statistically significant negative change; + = nonsignificant positive change; – = nonsignificant negative change; 0 = no change or conflicting results after move to community. From "Behavioral Outcomes of Deinstitutionalization of People With Intellectual Disabilities: A Review of U.S. Studies Conducted Between 1980 and 1999," by S. Kim, S. Larson, & K. C. Lakin, 2001, *Journal of Intellectual and Developmental Disabilities, 26,* pp. 40–43. Copyright 2001 by the Australian Society for the Study of Intellectual Disability, Inc. Adapted with permission of the Australian Society for the Study of Intellectual Disability, Inc

*scores not tested for statistical significance

and movements to the community than between movement to community and improvement in maladaptive behavior is an interesting phenomenon. It may be a result of the relatively more direct correspondence between the skills taught in normal community life and the skills measured in adaptive behavior than is the case with maladaptive behavior. Another factor may be the number of people with MR-DD who have psychiatric conditions that further complicate their learning of positive social behavior whether they live in institutions or in the community.

A recently published Norwegian study (Notlestad & Linaker, 1999) shows remarkable stability in psychiatric problems among people who had psychiatric disturbances before being released from institutions. The vast majority of sample members retained their diagnoses and associated problems after their movement to the community. Interestingly, although the psychiatric diagnosis of the individuals did not change, the frequency of measured challenging behavior among subjects increased in the areas of aggressive and disruptive behavior and in "passivity." The authors conclude that "Deinstitutionalization has not been shown to solve any problems connected with the mental health of people with intellectual disability" (p. 528).

Individual Rights and Equality of Opportunity

The *Olmstead* Decision

In the past three decades, all states have undertaken efforts to develop the accommodative capacity of their communities. The rates of development have, however, varied dramatically from state to state. Between 1990 and 1999, all 50 states decreased state institution populations, but the rate of decrease varied from 100% in 8 states that closed all state facilities of 15 or more residents to less than 25% in 9 states. Similarly, in 1999 three quarters (77%) of all residential service recipients lived in the community in settings of 15 or fewer residents; in 16 states the proportion was over 90%, but in 8 states still less than 60%.

Clearly most states have made substantial progress toward assuring community lives for all citizens with MR-DD, but others have much more to do. Consequently the primary determinant of people having access to opportunities and services that can support them, as needed, in the communities in which they live are their states and communities in which they have the fortune or misfortune to live. Arguing that restrictions that derive from government's unwillingness to respond to established benefits of community life, as identified and assured in the Americans With Disabilities Act (ADA; 1990), constituted unlawful discrimination, two individuals in Georgia used the civil rights protections under the ADA to pursue their desire for a place in the community. In June 1999 the Supreme Court of the United States issued a ruling, in *Olmstead et al. v. L.C. et al.,* of great potential significance to people with MR-DD who are or might be institutionalized. The *Olmstead v. L.C.* case tested the findings and purpose that Congress articulated in the ADA. Specifically, Congress noted in the ADA that the isolation and segregation of individuals with disabilities represented a "serious and pervasive social problem" because it was a form of discrimination (42 U.S.C. § 12101[a][2]), and that such discrimination was reflected in "outright intentional exclusion" and "relegation to lesser services, programs, activities, benefits, jobs, or other opportunities" (42 U.S.C. § 12101[a][5]). Congress noted that "the Nation's proper goals regarding individuals with disabilities are to assure equality of opportunity, full participation, independent living, economic self-sufficiency for such individuals" (42 U.SC. § 12101[a][8]). (See U.S. Equal Opportunity Commission, 1991, for the law, regulations, and interpretive guidance.)

The federal regulations (Title II — General Prohibition Against Discrimination, 1991), responding to the intent of Congress, required that a "public entity shall administer services, programs and activities in the most integrated setting appropriate to the needs of qualified individuals with disabilities" (28 C.F.R. § 35.130(d)). In considering *Olmstead* (1999), the Supreme Court reviewed whether the seemingly simple and clear language of the ADA actually prohibited a state from providing services to individuals with disabilities in an unnecessarily segregated setting and whether such mandate was violated when the state confines an individual with a disability in an institutionalized setting when a community setting is determined to be appropriate. Specifically the Court considered whether it was a violation of the ADA (i.e., was discrimination on the basis of describing) for a state to deny individuals community placement when community services were available to others, when community services were recommended for the individuals by the state's professionals, and when community services were desired by the individuals.

The majority opinion of the Court concluded that states are required to place individuals with mental disabilities in community settings rather than institutions when the state's treatment professionals have determined that a community placement is appropriate, the transfer is not opposed by the individual, and the placement can be reasonably accommodated given the resources available to the state and the needs of others with mental disabilities. In that opinion Justice Ginsberg noted:

> In the ADA, Congress not only required all public entities to refrain from discrimination . . . Congress explicitly identifies unjustified "segregation" of persons with disabilities as a "form of discrimination." . . . Recognition of unjustified segregation of persons with disabilities as a form of discrimination reflects two evident judgements. First, institutional placement of persons who can handle and benefit from community setting perpetuates unwarranted assumptions that persons so isolated are incapable and unworthy of participating in community life . . . Second, con-

finement in an institution severely diminishes the everyday life activities of individuals including family relations, social contacts, work options, economic independence, educational advancement, and cultural enrichment. (*Olmstead v. L.C.,* p. 596)

The significance of *Olmstead v. L. C.* (1999) is yet to be determined. It is likely to be most influential in states that have made the least progress in deinstitutionalization, but its implications are by no means limited to such states. It will contribute to the ongoing push to reduce institutionalization and to challenge communities to serve people who in the past have been viewed as appropriately housed in institutions.

A January 2000 letter to state Medicaid directors from the U.S. Departments of Health and Human Services and Justice noted that "This decision confirms what this Administration already believes: that no one should have to live in an institution or nursing home if they can live in the community with the right support" and that "*Olmstead* challenges states to prevent and correct inappropriate institutionalization and to review intake and admission processes to assure that people with disabilities are served in the most integrated setting appropriate" (Westmoreland & Perez, 2000, pp. 1–2).

Relevance of *Olmstead* to Behavioral Support or Crisis Response Programs
The fact the petitioners in *Olmstead* (1999) were people with histories of behavioral and psychiatric diagnoses and treatment is not insignificant. Over the past 20 years, as it has been recognized that severity of intellectual impairment is not an impediment to community life. As a consequence state institution populations of people with the most severe ("profound") intellectual disabilities have been reduced more than 50% (Anderson, Lakin, Prouty, & Polister, 1999). At the same time the use of institutions as a placement for people with behavioral and psychiatric disorders and MR-DD has become more common. In June 1998, 165 state institutions (84.2% of 197 total) reported that 41.4% of their residents had behavior disorders requiring special staffing, and 34.3% had psychiatric conditions requiring the involvement of professionals with psychiatric training (Anderson et al., 1999). *Olmstead* (1999) suggests that continued reliance on institutional settings as a primary locus for specialized services for people who present challenges to the community service system will be under growing pressure. It will no longer be acceptable to define a public or other type of institution as a designated or preferred place for treating behavioral and psychiatric disabilities. *Olmstead* suggests that specialized behavioral treatment capacities and responsibilities can no longer be concentrated in segregated settings when such services can be provided in the community with equal effectiveness and affordability. It further suggests that traditional uses of larger institutions as the "safety net" for emergencies and crises will be susceptible to challenges as less-segregating community alternatives are designed and demonstrated effective (Colond & Wieseler, 1995; Rudolph, Lakin,

Oslund, & Larson, 1998). As the aforementioned letter to Medicaid directors notes, "the requirement to provide services in the most integrated setting appropriate applies not only to people in institutional settings but to those being assessed for possible institutionalization" (Westmoreland & Perez, 2000, p. 2).

As (a) the *Olmstead v. L. C.* (1999) decision, (b) the advancing state-of-the-art in providing community services, and (c) the accomplishments of "institution-free" states challenge all states to provide community services to a wider range of people with MR-DD, the biggest challenge for most states is to develop and sustain effective behavioral support and crisis response services. For many states this will be difficult for several reasons: (a) they have focused their behavioral support resources and personnel in institutions; (b) they and their private contractors may have come to view these institutions as the "appropriate" places for people who present behavioral challenges; (c) state and private community agencies have often mutually accepted the institutions' offer of a place to send people with challenging behavior when they become difficult for community agencies to serve; (d) as a result of limited involvement in some states and among some service providers in responding to highly challenging and crisis behavior in the community, they have limited technical and experiential capacity to do so. The finding that an estimated 55.7% of 3,003 admissions to state institutions in FY 1998 were people with mild or moderate mental retardation and that 35.2% were people with mild mental retardation (c.f., an overall institutional population, 82.9% with severe and profound mental retardation) suggests a growing increasing use of state institutions for functions other than long-term care of people with severe cognitive impairments, frequently behavioral and psychiatric treatment (Anderson et al., 1999).

As demonstrated in the studies in Table 1.1, there is no evidence to support that institutional services are superior to community services in contributions to behavioral improvement. Community placement is increasingly recognized as the sine qua non of appropriate and effective services, yet those same studies show that it does not follow that community placement is sufficient to assure adequate, effective, and efficient responses to challenging behavior. To provide such responses states and agencies must carefully design delivery approaches for community behavioral supports that meet the needs of the individuals, service providers, and communities that they are to support.

The Importance of Community Capacity in Reducing Use of Institutions

Behavioral patterns and episodes that are difficult to manage in one's current environment, whether hurtful to others, hurtful to self, destructive of property, or disruptive of normal life, have been documented to jeopardize opportunities for

integrated community life. Research has shown that patterns of challenging behavior restrict people's opportunities for admission into community residential
and vocation programs (Hill et al., 1989; Scheerenberger, 1981). Challenging behavior has been the most consistently identified predictor of people's removal
from community programs and admission to institutional settings (Intagliata &
Willer, 1982; Lakin, Hill, Hauber, Bruininks, & Heal, 1983; Landesman-Dwyer
& Sultzbacher, 1981). As a result, higher prevalences of challenging behavior have
been found in institutional settings than in community environments (Bothwick-
Duffy, Eyman, & White, 1987; Hill & Bruininks, 1984; Lakin, Hill, Chen, &
Stephens, 1989).

Their challenging behavior has deprived people of opportunities to live in
community settings; if people do live in the community, such behavior, if unsuccessfully responded to, limits opportunities to participate in the community. People exhibiting challenging behavior have fewer social relationships with other
community members (Anderson, Lakin, Hill, & Chen, 1992; Larson, 1991).
They have fewer opportunities to participate in the community activities (Hill &
Bruininks, 1984). One nationwide study of the most integrated of residential
community settings (with six or fewer residents) found that residents who also had
significant levels of challenging behavior participated in fewer leisure activities in
their homes and fewer activities in their communities than people with lower rates
of problem behavior (Larson, 1991).

In many cases the lower rates of community participation result from staff
being viewed as inadequate to take someone with poorly controlled behavior into
settings where behavior is difficult to manage, where episodes of challenging behavior are highly disruptive or potentially damaging, and where stimuli that may
be associated with challenging behavior are most difficult to anticipate, avoid, or
eliminate. Beyond the implications to people's social lives, research suggests that
people with challenging behavior also are less likely to receive basic health services,
receiving fewer hours of dental services and therapy services than peers with lower
rates of challenging behavior (Hewitt, Larson, & Lakin, 2000; Jacobson, Silver, &
Schwartz, 1984).

A number of community behavioral support and crisis response programs
have been created in recent years to address the needs of individuals with developmental disabilities who display challenging behavior (Beasley, Kroll, & Sovner,
1992; Colond & Wieseler, 1995; Davidson et al., 1995). Those designing and
evaluating such programs have noted the importance of attending to mental
health problems. Given the high comorbidity of developmental disabilities and
psychiatric disorders and the significant potential for the misdiagnosis of psychiatric problems (Marcos, Gil, & Vasquez, 1986; Menolascino, Alberelli, & Gray,
1989; Reiss, 1990; Woodward, 1993), most existing models include mental
health professionals. Models for the provision of crisis services stress interdiscipli-

nary approaches, including treatment teams that incorporate psychiatric expertise (Beasley, Kroll, & Sovner, 1992) and links with the mental health system at both primary and tertiary levels (Davidson et al., 1995).

Existing community behavioral and crisis service program models have also emphasized prevention of behavioral crisis and/or short-term institutionalization. Colond and Wieseler (1995) documented the effectiveness of providing such services within the context of individuals' existing community residences. Davidson et al. (1995) stressed the early identification of individuals potentially at risk of needing crisis services and training for those individuals, their families, and service providers. Rudolph, Lakin, Oslund, and Larson (1998) demonstrated that the ability to prevent crises that culminate in institutional placement is the key to the cost effectiveness of behavioral support and crisis response services. Effective preventative approaches emphasize developing the crisis management capacity within organizations and identifying and developing the general skills of positive behavioral supports among community service providers and families (Beasley, Kroll, & Sovner, 1992; Davidson et al., 1995).

Designing, Evaluating, and Expanding Community Supports in Minnesota

The Special Services Program Demonstration

In 1992 the Minnesota state legislature authorized the demonstration of a community behavioral support and crisis response program to be housed in a vacated residential unit of Mount Olivet Rolling Acres. The purpose of this Special Services Program (SSP) was to establish community services and short-term crisis placements to eliminate the need for institutionalization. The legislature further required a quality and cost-effectiveness evaluation of the SSP outcomes. These outcomes were described in a report to the legislature (Rudolph & Lakin, 1995) and later summarized in an article published in *Mental Retardation* (Rudolph et al., 1998).

A total of 76 people were served by the SSP in its initial 19 months of operation. All of these people had lost or were considered at high risk of losing their current community home and being placed in a MR-DD, psychiatric, or correctional unit. Of the various presenting behavioral complaints of referred individuals, 70% involved aggression toward others or property destruction. Ten percent of the complaints were for forms of self-injurious behavior, 12% for running away or other noncompliance. Six percent were for criminal acts other than assault or property destruction (i.e., theft and unlawful sexual behavior). Among the general outcomes of the program were universal satisfaction from primary caregivers of the individuals referred (56% "very high," 44% "high"). Service coordinators of the referred individuals also reported universal satisfaction (63% "very high," 37%

"high"). Despite general satisfaction, case managers expressed concern about the 90-day crisis-unit limit; alternative placements or current placement enhancements were difficult to achieve in the allotted time. Over the course of the demonstration, only one person was admitted to a state institution subsequent to participation in the program. That institutional placement occurred because of a decision to enforce the 90-day limit on crisis-unit placements despite the absence of an alternative placement at the end of that period. Subsequent to the evaluation of the initial program, a transition placement option was created; this maintained commitment to a 90-day maximum "crisis placement" but permitted longer than 90 days to complete the individualized planning and service development needed to meet unique characteristics and needs of some program participants.

An extensive evaluation of the cost-effectiveness of achieving the outcomes showed the SSP was able to support, provide, and develop community services to prevent institutionalization at about 60% of the estimated costs of the services that would have been provided in the absence of the SSP. The estimates were based on information from service coordinators of 54 people referred to SSP over 1 year; they were asked to develop, based on their experience, what would be the most likely scenarios for these individuals had the new SSP services not been available. Each scenario was then priced out based on actual average expenditures and service days for the "projected" scenarios. Based on these projections, the additional crisis-related expenditures for the 54 individuals in the SSP demonstration were estimated to be more than $720,000 or $13,400 per person. These projected additional expenditures over 1 year were $287,000 more than the actual cost of the SSP ($435,150) and in the process kept a projected 27 people from being admitted to state institutions and 7 more out of psychiatric units. The "projections" of the service coordinators of the 54 individuals were validated through follow-up studies of 14 individuals who were referred to, but could not be served in, the SSP demonstration because of limitations on SSP capacity and because of their residence outside the SSP catchment area. Service coordinators had projected that 27 of the 54 referrals (50%) would have been placed in a state institution; 7 of the 14 members of the validation group (50%) were actually placed in a state institution. In all, 11 of the 14 (78.6%) in the validation group were placed outside the home in which they were living at the time of their referral (to state institutions, psychiatric units, congregate care settings). This compared with projections of 43 of 54 (79.6%) by service coordinators for the SSP referrals. In these and other ways, the potential cost-effectiveness of community-based crisis response and behavioral support programs was established, but it was also recognized that creating alternatives to state institutional placements could contribute to systemwide cost effectiveness if the services for which they could be substituted (i.e., state institutions) actually ceased to expend resources.

Planning an All-Community Future

In the period subsequent to the development of Special Services Program, behavior support and crisis response programs offering direct services, consultation, and resource coordination were implemented to include catchment areas serving a substantial majority of individuals with MR-DD in Minnesota. As a product of this commitment, the last of Minnesota's state MR-DD institutions closed in the year 2000, although the state still maintains the Minnesota Extended Treatment Options for court-ordered treatment or custody of about 40 people. A great deal of planning and coordination was required and continues to be carried out to allow Minnesotans with MR-DD to receive the behavioral and crisis support they sometimes need without the "back-up" of public institutions.

In the early 1990s, it was clear that Minnesota was moving steadily and irreversibly toward the day when few if any people with MR-DD would be living in state institutions. Between June 1990, when Minnesota had about 1,350 residents in seven state institutions, and June 1995, residents decreased by over 60% to just over 500 (while per person costs increased by 60%).

So already by 1993 and 1994, it was apparent that the policy decisions had been already made that would make closing all Minnesota's public institutions inevitable. The challenge to Minnesotans was to plan for a rapidly approaching future that would only in 4 years bring the state institution populations down to 68 people in two institutions (at an average cost of $615 per day) and would by June 2000 lead to closure of all of Minnesota's state institutions for people with MR-DD, except for the aforementioned Minnesota Extended Treatment Options.

Planning for that rapidly approaching future included developing and testing alternative community services like the SSP. It also meant anticipating and attempting to accommodate growing complexities. For example, from about 1,800 total residential settings in 1991 it was projected that the number of residential settings for people with MR-DD would double by 1999 and that more than 6,000 people would be receiving support services in their family homes (actual numbers in June 1999 were 3,500 in residential settings and 7,200 individuals served while living with their families). Unknown thousands of other children and adults with MR-DD continued to reside with their natural or adoptive families while attending school or working in their communities, and, although not then service recipients, many were separated from the formal service system only by a single episode or crisis. Developing a system of behavioral support and crisis response to address these growing complexities and potential demands for services was an organizational challenge.

Defining Alternatives to the Institutional "Safety Net"

As Minnesota was rapidly decreasing its institutional capacity so as to better respond to the human development, dignity, and rights of its citizens, it was becoming increasingly clear that Minnesota's institutions existed almost exclusively to serve as a general "safety net" for individuals with very challenging behavior, people under criminal commitment, people experiencing severe behavioral or emotional crisis, and/or people who needed an immediate place to go. Upon analysis, it was clear that Minnesota's institutions' only valued systematic function was that of an ever-ready, immediate placement of last resort for people with extensive behavioral needs or for those experiencing other forms of crisis. Longitudinal analysis of admissions showed that, despite a nearly two-thirds reduction in state institution populations between 1985 and 1994, because of these systemic functions, overall admissions had changed very little. Average annual admissions had decreased only from 168 in 1985–1986 to 154 in 1993–1994. But most of these admissions (77%) were "short-term" (90 or fewer days), suggesting that problems were soluble within the home or community.

Developing a Community-Support System

In 1994 a "working group" of Minnesota stakeholders, including representatives of state and local government, private agencies, advocacy organizations, consumers, and families, began to plan a design for a system of Behavioral Support and Crisis Response for Minnesotans With Developmental Disabilities (Lakin & Rudolph, 1995). This design proposal, bolstered by documentation of the outcomes of the SSP demonstration, contributed to legislation in 1995 authorizing a statewide network of programs of community-based crisis services for people with developmental disabilities. By far the largest and most fully developed of these programs is in the Metro Crisis Coordination Program (MCCP). MCCP was developed by Mount Olivet Rolling Acres (MORA), which also administers the SSP. MCCP coordinates crisis services in the Minneapolis-St. Paul metropolitan area, a seven-county area that contains 53% of Minnesota's population.

Referrals

Referrals usually come to MCCP from county social services agencies, often in response to caregiver request. MCCP takes cases that are not expected to need more than 90 days of service. Individuals who have need for longer-term intervention are typically referred to a state-operated community support services (CSS) team, SSP, or other specialist agencies.

Reasons for referral to MCCP include an immediate crisis, a request for preventative services, or requests for information and/or referral. A crisis may be caused by situational, behavioral, or medical factors, including when a caregiver is overwhelmed, ill, or otherwise unable to provide care, when an individual's behavior becomes dangerous to self or others, or when the person's crisis is related to the need for medication monitoring or adjustment. Requests for preventive services are usually made by service coordinators when there is a concern that caregivers may be losing their ability to manage a situation adequately or safely. Information and referral requests are received from service coordinators, family members, or others who need information about services or other crisis resources.

Services
MCCP responds within 24 hours to crisis calls. During business hours, MCCP may be reached directly, and an answering machine is used for after-business hours. After-hour calls for emergencies are given a number that pages an on-call MCCP staff member. MCCP behavior analysts respond to emergency calls and attempt to stabilize the situation and ensure that it is safe. They assess the situation, generally at the client's place of residence, school, or day program, interview caregivers, and observe to determine the best course of action. Training and technical assistance are provided by MCCP staff to support family members and staff at the residence and work, school, or day program. MCCP also maintains a statewide list of all residential openings and related service capacities for people with developmental disabilities.

Users
Between March 1998 and September 1999, MCCP received 676 crisis referrals. MCCP provided technical assistance in 263 (39%) cases classified as "preventative" and 247 (36%) cases classified as "emergency." In addition, MCCP provided information and referral service to 166 cases (25%). Of the total 676 cases, 30% involved individuals with whom MCCP had previously been involved in some capacity. All but 11 (2%) of the individuals whom MCCP served during this time had a mental retardation diagnoses: 388 (57%) mild, 147 (22%) moderate, 82 (12%) severe, 35 (5%) profound, and 13 (2%) undetermined. (This distribution is quite different than the distribution of Minnesotans with MR-DD in the state intermediate care facilities for people with mental retardation (ICF-MR) and home and community-based services ("waiver") programs: 29% mild, 26% moderate, 22% severe, 22% profound, and 0.2 % undetermined).

At the time of MCCP referral, 223 (33%) individuals lived with their family, 244 (36%) lived in Medicaid home and community-based services (HCBS) waiver-financed settings, 65 (10%) lived in ICF-MRs, 60 (9%) in foster care, 8 (1%) were in hospitals, 6 (1%) were in criminal justice facilities, 5 (1%) were living in their own homes, and 65 (10%) were recorded as "other."

Staff

MCCP staff members include an operational coordinator, a clinical coordinator, seven behavior analysts, a psychiatric nurse, and an office manager who also is responsible for the intake process. The operational coordinator is responsible for administration, marketing, and creating links with hospitals and other service providers. He also manages a caseload of six to eight preventative cases. The clinical coordinator is responsible for the supervision and oversight of the outreach workers' clinical work and carries an 80% to 90% caseload. Six of the behavior analysts carry an average of 10 to 12 cases. Behavior analysts conduct functional assessments and make recommendations for plans of care (crisis plans and behavior plans). They also provide technical assistance to caregivers and support staff. A seventh behavior analyst has primary responsibility for information and referral and housing issues and shares preventative cases with the operational coordinator. The full-time psychiatric nurse assists in coordinating hospital services, admissions, and discharges, and provides consultation to MCCP staff on health and medication concerns. MCCP also pays part of the salary for a psychiatric nurse and behavior analyst at SSP and uses them on an as-needed basis.

Case Example: Emily

Emily, age 46, has lived in institutional settings from the time she was 9 years old. At the time of her referral to MCCP, Emily was living in a group home of 11 residents. Her diagnoses include severe mental retardation with pica behavior. She has no family involvement; even so, she has experienced high levels of stability in her direct support staff and her service coordinator. In the past 5 years, Emily has had two crises to which the SSP responded.

Emily was referred to MCCP because of her pica (ingesting mouthwash, jewelry, and urine) and for self-injury through pushing sticks up her nose and picking and biting herself to the point of drawing blood. She was also noted less frequently to pinch, push, hit, pull hair, and take things of others. MCCP was contacted as Emily's problem behaviors were increasing at home and work; her present team saw the increases as deserving outside assessment; they perceived that a new living arrangement if properly planned could help improve Emily's life and behavior.

An MCCP staff member conducted the requested assessment and developed interventions and training for direct support staff around the pica behavior. He helped develop planned interventions around the decision made with Emily, her interdisciplinary team, and service provider that a smaller, quieter setting would probably be helpful to Emily. He worked with residential and vocational service providers to coordinate the planned interventions and to assure common understanding of Emily's signals and other communication. He continued to follow up with both the residential and vocational agencies and to make plan modifications with them based on the relative success of the different components of the plan.

Emily's pica, self-injury, and aggressive behavior decreased significantly following MCCP referral. No particular attributions are made about the success. All people involved believe that Emily's move to a very different new environment was very important to her, as was the supported attention to her more positive behavior. For Emily's support staff and service coordinator, the important aspects of MCCP involvement were that (a) the plans developed were simple and could be implemented within the context and demands of their role; (b) MCCP identified what was not working, offered modifications and "fine-tuning" of original plans, and continued to stay engaged; (c) MCCP provided a link and means to develop consistency in the understanding of and response to Emily across residential and vocational sites; and (d) MCCP reinforced the good efforts of caring staff working in what was often a difficult and stressful circumstance.

In sum, what was most valued in Emily's situation and in most of those in other case studies in the MCCP evaluation was not the skills and astuteness of MCCP staff. The skills and expertise are appreciated, but support staff and service coordinators appreciate even more the MCCP commitment to get and stay involved in situations that seldom have easy or quick answers and for which there is no longer the alternative of sending "the problem" off to a state institution. (See Bast, Constantine, & Lakin, 1999, for other brief case studies.)

Lessons of the Minnesota Experience

The past 8 years of effort to develop community behavior support and crisis response programs in Minnesota and the concurrent commitment to closing Minnesota's state institutions have taught some basic lessons. These lessons have guided the continued evolution of behavioral support crisis response services in Minnesota. They have also provided the general themes around which this volume has been organized. These themes included:

Recognize the High Costs of Inaction

In the long term, it had to be recognized in Minnesota that if state institution depopulation continued in the absence of community alternatives for behavioral support and crisis response, the system would eventually experience very large increases in service expenditures and/or human costs. Such costs would be incurred through requiring the maintenance of state MR-DD institutions as a "safety net" (in the last FY Minnesota's state institutions have had average per person expenditures of $615 per day) and/or there would be increasingly high costs through greater dependence on psychiatric facility admissions and longer lengths of stay at huge expenditures (an average about $1,000 per day) to meet behavior support needs. Denial of access to behavioral supports led to injury, homelessness, emotional impairment, and other unacceptable outcomes.

Establish a Foundation of Efficiency and Acceptability
As people began to consider ways to expand the benefits of the earlier demonstration to broader audiences and geographics, they looked at important political and economic considerations. It was important to recognize, value, and include in the planning process people with high stakes in and capacity to contribute to a noninstitutional approach to behavioral support. It was equally important to appreciate that all participants had insights, skills, and commitments to offer.

Base Programs on Valid and Accepted Treatment Principles
Challenging behavior and behavioral crises are the product of a wide range of interactions between people with MR-DD and their social environments. An effective system would need to address a wide array of circumstances and needs, including not only those amenable to traditional behavioral analysis, but also, and more often, those requiring social-environmental changes, physical-medical assessment and treatment, communication development and augmentation, new ways of planning around specific personal preferences, and other responses to circumstances that may underlie challenging behavior and resulting crisis. To provide a full range of needed responses, it is important that a comprehensive, evaluated treatment approach be adopted, and that people involved in the various components of the community receive comprehensive and conceptually congruent initial and ongoing training.

Be Responsive to Key Consumers
An effective behavioral support and crisis response program must operate in a supportive partnership with the individuals, families, counties, private and public providers, mental health providers, state agency representatives, and communities being served. This involves (a) obtaining feedback and guidance from its service users and funders, (b) engaging in ongoing identification of the individual and collective needs of key consumers, (c) monitoring successes and shortcomings in meeting those needs, (d) identifying existing and needed resources and expertise to be responsive to people needs, and (e) establishing ways to develop or obtain access to new resources and services as needed. It means ongoing independent evaluation, but, more important, ongoing review of services with consumers, direct support staff, service coordinators, families, and others.

Integrate Existing Resources and Expertise
In developing community supports, professional, economic, and political realities required integration of the resources, expertise, and experience of the state-operated Community Supports Services, the Special Services Program, and other specialized programs and professionals. Such programs and their staffs provided an excellent foundation of experience for expanding access to services, but we recognized that

integrating them into a definable program with a single point of entry, a common approach, quality control, and common expectations would be an initial and on-going challenge.

Change the Culture of "Easy Out"

When public institutions functioned as places to send people who presented behavioral challenges, it became convenient for private service providers to take advantage of that function. Operating without public institutions and with a very limited "crisis bed capacity" requires that service providers stay engaged and work with behavioral support staff to respond effectively to people who once would have been remanded to the state institution. The establishment of a program of skilled practitioners who exhibit a commitment to stay engaged, and who build on a foundation of effectiveness in previous efforts have helped create a new level of commitment of service providers to endure and effectively respond to the challenges of those they serve.

Stay on the "Side" of People With Disabilities

Many of the challenges in providing behavioral support and crisis response services derive from a serious mismatch between people and their environments. Too much of the history of behavioral treatment has focused on how to induce conformity to a "given" environment. Interventions with potential for long-term positive outcomes often require sufficient respect and skill to listen to individuals to understand and appreciate the extent to which their daily lives reflect their own personal goals, needs, and desires. Long-term positive outcomes often require the honesty to recognize the inadequacies of the existing circumstances, commitment to make the changes needed to make people's lives better, and the options and creativity to help people build lives that better reflect what they want and need.

This book describes the design and implementation approaches incorporating these and other lessons learned in efforts to support people with intellectual and developmental disabilities. In presenting their knowledge and experiences, the authors offer substantial hope that with appropriate community support all people with intellectual and developmental disabilities can be and can remain residents of homes and neighborhoods in typical communities.

References

Abery, B. H., & Fahnestock, M. (1994). Enhancing the social inclusion of persons with developmental disabilities. In M. F. Hayden & B. H. Abery (Eds.), *Challenges for a service system in transition: Ensuring quality community experiences for persons with developmental disabilities* (pp. 83–119). Baltimore: Paul H. Brookes.

Abery, B. H., Thurlow, M. T., Johnson, D. R., & Bruininks, R. H. (1990, May). *The social networks of adults with developmental disabilities residing in community settings.* Paper presented at the annual meeting of the American Association on Mental Retardation, Washington, DC.

Americans With Disabilities Act of 1990, 42 U.S.C.A. § 12101 *et seq.* (West 1993).

Anderson, D. J., Lakin, K. C., Hill, B. K., & Chen, T. H. (1992). Social integration of older persons in residential facilities. *American Journal on Mental Retardation, 96*(5), 488–501.

Anderson, L., Lakin, K. C., Prouty, R., & Polister, B. (1999). Characteristics and movement of residents of large state facilities. In R. Prouty & K. C. Lakin (Eds.), *Residential services for persons with developmental disabilities: Status and trends through 1998.* Minneapolis: University of Minnesota, Research and Training Center on Community Living, Institute on Community Integration.

Apgar, D. H., Cook, S., & Lerman, P. (1998). *Life after Johnstone: Impacts on consumer competencies, behaviors, and quality of life.* Newark: New Jersey Institute of Technology, Center for Architecture and Building Science Research.

Bast, J., Constantine, M., & Lakin, K. C. (1999). *Perspectives on the use and users of the Metro Crisis Coordination Program.* Minneapolis: University of Minnesota, Research and Training Center on Community Living, Institute on Community Integration.

Beasley, J., Kroll, J., & Sovner, R. (1992). Community-based crisis mental health services for persons with developmental disabilities: The START model. *Habilitative Mental Health Newsletter, 11,* 55–57.

Bolin, B. L. (1994). *Developmental disabilities quality assurance: A study of deinstitutionalization.* Unpublished doctoral dissertation, Oklahoma State University, Stillwater.

Borthwick-Duffy, S., Eyman, R., & White, J. (1987). Client characteristics and residential placement patterns. *American Journal of Mental Deficiency of Mental Deficiency, 92*(1), 24–30.

Braddock, D., Hemp, R., Parish, S., & Rizzolo, M. (2000). *The state of the states in developmental disabilities: 2000 study summary.* Chicago: University of Illinois at Chicago, Department of Disability and Human Development.

Braddock, D., Hemp, R., Parish, S., & Westrich, J. (1998). *The state of the states in developmental disabilities* (5th ed.). Washington, DC: American Association of Mental Retardation.

Bradley, V. J., Conroy, J. W., Covert, S. B., & Feinstein, C. S. (1986). *Community Options: The New Hampshire choice.* Cambridge, MA: Human Services Research Institute.

Business Services Group. (1999). *Longitudinal quality of life study: Phase III.* Sacramento: California State University, Sacramento, Business Services Group.

Calapai, P. (1988). *Adaptive behaviors of developmentally disabled adults living in community residences.* Unpublished doctoral dissertation. Hofstra University, Hempstead, NY.

Center for Outcome Analysis. (1999). *The Indiana Quality Tracking Project on DC closures: Preliminary findings.* Bryn Mawr, PA: Author.

Close, D. W. (1977). Community living for severely and profoundly retarded adults: A group home study. *Education and Training of the Mentally Retarded, 12,* 256–262.

Colond, J. S., & Wieseler, N. A. (1995). Preventing restrictive placements through community support services. *American Journal on Mental Retardation, 100*(3), 201–206.

Colorado Division of Developmental Disabilities. (1982). *Colorado's regional center satellite group homes: An evaluation report.* Denver: Author.

Conroy, J. W. (1995). *The Hissom outcome study: A report on six years of movement into supported living. The well-being of people with developmental disabilities in Oklahoma* (Brief Rep. No. 1). Ardmore, PA: Center for Outcome Analysis.

Conroy, J. W. (1998). *Are people better off? Outcomes of the closure of Winfield State Hospital.* Report submitted to the Kansas Council on Developmental Disabilities. Rosemont, PA: Center for Outcome Analysis.

Conroy, J. W., & Bradley, V. J. (1985). *The Pennhurst longitudinal study: A report of five years of research and analysis.* Philadelphia: Temple University, Developmental Disabilities Center. Boston: Human Services Research Institute.

Conroy, J., Efthimiou, J., & Lemanowicz, J. (1982). A matched comparison of the developmental growth of institutionalized and deinstitutionalized mentally retarded clients. *American Journal of Mental Deficiency, 86,* 581–587.

Conroy, J. W., Feinstein, C. S., & Lemanowicz, J. A. (1988). *Results of the longitudinal study of* CARC v. Thorne *class members* (Rep. No. 7). Philadelphia: Temple University, Developmental Disabilities Center.

Conroy, J. W., Lemanowicz, J. A., Feinstein, C. S., & Bernotsky, J. M. (1991). *1990 results of the* CARC v. Thorne *longitudinal study. The Connecticut Applied Research Project* (Rep. No. 10). Narberth, PA: Conroy & Feinstein Associates.

Conroy, J. W., Seiders, J., & Yuskauskas, A. (1998). *Patterns of community placement IV: The fourth annual report on the outcomes of implementing the Coffelt settlement agreement* (Rep. No. 17). Bryn Mawr, PA: Center for Outcome Analysis.

D'Amico, M. L., Hannah, M. A., Milhouse, J. A., & Froleich, A. K. (1978). *Evaluation of adaptive behavior. Institutional vs. community placements and treatment for the mentally retarded.* Stillwater: Oklahoma State University, National Clearing House of Rehabilitation Materials.

Davidson, P., Cain, N., Sloan-Reeves, J., Giesow, V., Quijano, L., VanHeyningen, J., & Shohan, I. (1995). Crisis intervention for community-based individuals with developmental disabilities and behavioral and psychiatric disorders. *Mental Retardation, 33,* 21–30.

Davis, V. J. (1990). *A follow-up study of the development of mentally retarded individuals placed in the community compared with a sample who remained in a residential center.* Unpublished doctoral dissertation, University of Pittsburgh, PA.

Eastwood, E. A. (1985). *Community living study: Three reports of client development, family impact, and the cost of services among community-based and institutionalized persons with mental retardation.* Belchertown, MA: Belchertown State School.

Eastwood, E. A., & Fisher, G. A. (1988). Skill acquisition among matched samples of institutionalized and community-based persons with mental retardation. *American Journal on Mental Retardation, 93,* 75–83.

Feinstein, C. S., Lemanowicz, J. A., Spreat, S., & Conroy, J. W. (1986). *Report to the special master in the case of* Gary W. v. the State of Louisiana. Philadelphia: Temple University, Developmental Disabilities Center.

Feinstein, C. S., Lemanowicz, J. A., & Conroy, J. W. (1988). *A survey of satisfaction with regional treatment centers and community services to persons with mental retardation in Minnesota.* Philadelphia: Conroy & Feinstein Associates.

Felce, D., de Kock, U., & Repp, A. C. (1986). An eco-behavioral analysis of small community-based houses and traditional large hospitals for severely and profoundly mentally handicapped adults. *Applied Research in Mental Retardation, 7,* 393–408.

Fortune, J., Heinlein, K. B., & Fortune, B. (1995). Changing the shape of the service population. *European Journal of Mental Disability, 2*(8), 20–37.

Fuess, B. (1987). *The past institutional adjustment of elderly mentally retarded and develomentally disabled persons: A population study.* Unpublished doctoral dissertation, Ohio State University.

Fujiura, G. T. (1998). Commentary on the meaning of residential mortality research. *Mental Retardation, 36*(5), 400–403.

Hayden, M. F., DePaepe, P., Soulen, T., & Polister, B. (1995). *Deinstitutionalization and community integration of adults with mental retardation: Summary and comparison of the baseline and one-year follow-up residential data for the Minnesota Longitudinal Study* (Project Rep. 1). Minneapolis: University of Minnesota, Research and Training Center on Community Living, Institute on Community Integration.

Hewitt, A., Larson, S. A., & Lakin, K. C. (2000). *An independent evaluation of the quality of services and system performance of Minnesota's Medicaid Home and Community Based Services for persons with mental retardation and related conditions* (Technical Rep.). Minneapolis: University of Minnesota, Research and Training Center on Community Living.

Hill, B. K., & Bruininks, R. H. (1984). Maladaptive behavior of mentally retarded people in residential facilities. *American Journal of Mental Deficiency, 88*(4), 380–387.

Hill, B. K., Lakin, K. C., Bruininks, R. H., Amado, A. N., Anderson, D. J., & Copher, J. I. (1989). *Living in the community: A comparative study of foster homes and small group homes for people with mental retardation.* Minneapolis: University of Minnesota, Research and Training Center on Community Living, Institute on Community Integration.

Horner, R. H., Stoner, S. K., & Ferguson, D. L. (1988). *An activity-based analysis of deinstitutionalization: The effects of community re-entry on the lives of residents leaving Oregon's Fairview Training Center.* Salem: University of Oregon, Specialized Training Center on Human Development.

Intagliata, J., & Willer, B. (1982). Reinstitutionalization of mentally retarded persons successfully placed into family-care and group homes. *American Journal of Mental Deficiency, 87*(1), 34–39.

Jacobson, J. W., Silver E., & Schwartz, A. (1984). Service provision in New York's group homes. *Mental Retardation, 22,* 231–239.

Kim, S., Larson, S., & Lakin, K. C. (2001). Behavioral outcomes of deinstitutionalization of people with intellectual disabilities: A review of U.S. studies conducted between 1980 and 1999. *Journal of Intellectual and Developmental Disability, 26*(1), 35–50.

Kleinberg, J., & Galligan, B. (1983). Effects of deinstitutionalization on adaptive behavior of mentally retarded adults. *American Journal of Mental Deficiency, 88,* 21–27.

Lakin, K. C., Anderson, L., & Prouty, R. W. (1998). Decreases continue in out-of-home placements of children and youth with mental retardation. *Mental Retardation, 36*(2), 165–168.

Lakin, K. C., Hill, B. K., & Bruininks, R. H. (1985) *An analysis of Medicaid's Intermediate Care Facility for the Mentally Retarded (ICF-MR) program.* Minneapolis: University of Minnesota, Research and Training Center on Community Living, Institute of Community Integration.

Lakin, K. C., Hill, B. K., Chen, T. H., & Stephens, S. A. (1989). *Persons with mental retardation and related conditions in mental retardation facilities: Selected findings from the 1987 National Medicaid Expenditures Survey.* Minneapolis: University of Minnesota, Research and Training Center on Community Living, Institute on Community Integration.

Lakin, K. C., Hill, B. K., Hauber, F. A., Bruininks, R. H., & Heal, L. W. (1983). New admissions and readmissions to a national sample of residential facilities. *American Journal of Mental Deficiency, 88,* 13–20.

Lakin, K. C., & Rudolph, C. (Eds). (1995, January). *A design for a system of behavioral support and crisis response for Minnesotans with developmental disabilities: Recommendations of the Working Group on Behavioral Support and Crisis Response.* Minneapolis: University of Minnesota, Research and Training Center on Community Living, Institute on Community Integration.

Landesman-Dwyer, S., & Sulzberger, F. M. (1981). Residential placement and adaptation of severely and profoundly retarded individuals. In R. Bruininks, C. Meyers, B. Sigford, & K. C. Lakin (Eds.), *Deinstitutionalization and community adjustment of mentally retarded people* (pp. 182–194). Washington, DC: American Association on Mental Deficiency.

Larson, S. A. (1991). Quality of Life for people with challenging behavior living in community settings. *IMPACT, 4*(1), 4–5.

Larson, S. A., & Lakin, K. C. (1989). Deinstitutionalization of persons with mental retardation: The impact on daily living skills. *Journal of The Association for Persons With Severe Handicaps, 14*(4), 324–332.

Larson, S. A., & Lakin, K. C. (1991). Parental attitudes about residential placement before and after deinstitutionalization: A research synthesis. *Journal of The Association for Persons With Severe Handicaps, 16,* 25–38.

Marcos, L., Gil, R., & Vasquez, K. (1986). Who will treat psychiatrically disturbed developmentally disabled patients? A health care nightmare. *Hospital and Community Psychiatry, 37,* 171–174.

Menolascino, F., Alberelli, M., & Gray, V. (1989). *Mental retardation and mental health: Classification, diagnosis, treatment, and services.* New York: Springer-Verlag.

Molony, H., & Taplin, J. E. (1990). The deinstitutionalization of people with developmental disability under the Richmond program: Changes in adaptive behavior. *Australia and New Zealand Journal of Developmental Disabilities, 16*(2), 149–159.

Notlestad, J., & Linaker, O. (1999). Psychiatric health needs and services before and after complete deinstitutionalization of people with intellectual disability. *Journal of Intellectual Disability Research, 43*(6), 523–530.

Olmstead v. L. C., 527 U.S. 581.596 (1999).

O'Neill, J., Brown, M., Gordon, W., & Schonhorn, R (1985). The impact of deinstitutionalization on activities and skills of severely/profoundly mentally retarded multiply-handicapped adults. *Applied Research in Mental Retardation, 6,* 361–371.

Prouty, R., & Lakin, K. C. (1999). *Residential services for persons with developmental disabilities: Status and trends through 1998.* Minneapolis: University of Minnesota, Research and Training Center on Community Living, Institute on Community Integration.

Prouty, R., Smith, G., & Lakin, K. C. (Eds.). (2001). *Residential services for persons with developmental disabilities: Status and trends through 2000.* Minneapolis: University of Minnesota, Research and Training Center on Community Living, Institute on Community Integration.

Reiss, S. (1990). Prevalence and dual diagnosis in community-based day programs in the Chicago metropolitan area. *American Journal on Mental Retardation, 94,* 578–585.

Rose, K. C., White, J. A., Conroy, J., & Smith, D. M. (1993). Following the course of a change: A study of adaptive and maladaptive behaviors in young adults living in the community. *Education and Training in Mental Retardation, 28*(2), 149–154.

Rosen, D. B. (1985). *Differences in adaptive behavior of institutionalized and deinstitutionalized mentally retarded adults.* Ann Arbor, MI. (University Microfilms International No. DA8508127)

Rudolf, C. & Lakin, K. C. (1995). *Final evaluation of the Mt. Olivet Rolling Acres Special Services Program.* Minneapolis: University of Minnesota, Research and Training Center on Community Living, Institute on Community Integration.

Rudolf, C., Lakin, K. C., Oslund, J. M., & Larson, W (1998). Evaluation of outcomes and cost effectiveness of a community behavioral support and crisis response demonstration project. *Mental Retardation, 36*(3), 187–197.

Scheerenberger, R. (1981). Deinstitutionalization: Trends and difficulties. In R. Bruininks, C. Meyers, B. Sigford, & K. C. Lakin (Eds.), *Deinstitutionalization and community adjustment of mentally retarded people* (pp. 3–13). Washington, DC: American Association on Mental Deficiency.

Schroeder, S. R., & Hanes, C. (1978). Assessment of progress of institutionalized and deinstitutionalized retarded adults: A matched-control comparison. *Mental Retardation, 16,* 147–148.

Stancliffe, R. J., & Lakin, K. C. (1998). Analysis of expenditures and outcomes of residential alternatives for persons with developmental disabilities. *American Journal on Mental Retardation, 103*(6), 552–568.

Thompson, T., & Carey, A. (1980). Structured normalization: Intellectual and adaptive behavior changes in a residential setting. *Mental Retardation, 18,* 193–197.

U.S. Equal Opportunity Commission, U.S. Department of Justice. (1991, December). *Americans With Disabilities Act Handbook.* (Washington, D.C.: U.S. Government Printing Office.)

Westmoreland, T. M., & Perez, T. (2000, January). *Dear Medicaid director.* [Online], Health Care Financing Administration. Available: www.hcfa.gov

Willer, B., & Intagliata, J. (1980). *Deinstitutionalization of mentally retarded persons in New York State.* Buffalo: State University of New York at Buffalo, Research Foundation.

Williams, B. W., Paskow, F. S., Thompson, L., & Levine, M. P. (1985). *The effects of deinstitutionalization on adaptive and maladaptive behaviors of mentally retarded persons.* Unpublished manuscript.

Woodward, H. (1993). One community's response to the multisystem service needs of individuals with mental illness and developmental disabilities. *Community Mental Health Journal, 29,* 347–359.

CHAPTER 2

The Challenges of Providing Behavioral Support and Crisis Response Services in the Community

Ronald H. Hanson
Mount Olivet Rolling Acres
Victoria, Minnesota

Norman A. Wieseler
Eastern Minnesota Community Support Services
Faribault, Minnesota

The deinstitutionalization of people with mental retardation or related conditions has produced dramatic changes to these individuals' lives. This was especially evident for those clients with aberrant patterns of challenging behaviors, such as aggression toward others, self-injury, property destruction, public disrobing, sexual predation, and other problematic behaviors that were previously managed within the institutional confines. Behavior programs and psychotropic medications have been the primary strategies for reducing the frequency and intensity of behavior disorders.

Once clients with histories of challenging behavior were transferred to community settings, problem behaviors dissipated for many; for some, behaviors increased; others remained unchanged.

There have been many untoward effects of people exhibiting challenging behaviors in the community. Some clients experienced emergency hospital admissions into psychiatric care units. Many clients lived with increased restrictions under more intensive supervision, while peers, without challenging behaviors, enjoyed greater community freedoms. When clients displayed severe problem behaviors that violated community standards, their integrated placements were terminated and they were returned to institutional settings.

To prevent the loss of community living, specialized services are required. Although advances in pharmacotherapy have resulted in fewer side effects in treating mental health disorders, additional behavioral services are generally required. These crisis prevention and response services should be conducted and monitored by professionals with expertise in the treatment of challenging behaviors using positive behavioral support and intervention.

As chapters in this monograph reveal, many states have developed crisis prevention and response services to address behavioral crises in the community. These support systems are enormously important for many clients at risk of losing the freedoms of community living. However, other states or regions have been to date ineffective in either the development or the actual provision of crisis services.

Influencing Forces

Many forces have been identified that influence the development and provision of crisis services. These include (a) litigation, (b) existing services provided by other units of government, (c) legislation responding to the wishes of family members and care providers, (d) current services provided by existing practitioners, (e) advocacy efforts, and (f) trade union agreements. In addition to these forces, the desire to spend Medicaid dollars more wisely has prompted some states to create crisis prevention and response services that enabled at-risk clients to remain in their community placements rather than relying on psychiatric hospitalizations.

Although for some clients, psychiatric hospitalization has been the only available treatment option, it often has proven disruptive and problematic, both for the client and staff of the community residence and the psychiatric hospital unit. The hospitalized patient with developmental disabilities can be vulnerable to exploitation by higher-functioning psychiatric patients, requiring very close supervision by hospital personnel. Hospital staff often have limited experience working with individuals with severe intellectual disabilities and, in some cases, have requested that the client's care providers remain present in the hospital throughout his or her hospital stay. While such extra staffing provides enhanced care, it can reduce the staff-client ratios at the client's home program. As a whole, the cost of providing specialized crisis prevention and response service is offset by the savings resulting from the avoidance of costly psychiatric hospitalizations.

Litigation

Many states have experienced litigation that forced, and then accelerated, the closure of their large state-operated facilities (e.g., California, see chap. 5, this volume). At the federal level, in the 1980s Senator John Chafee (1988) introduced

Medicaid reform legislation specifically focused on downsizing large congregate care facilities. According to Scheerenberger (1983), the federal courts took a major interest in institutions and examined constitutionally the care that was, or was not, being provided. The first case to address the constitutional right to treatment was *Wyatt v. Stickney* (1972). The judge in this case found that the Alabama Department on Mental Hygiene had violated the constitutional rights of the mentally retarded residents. He specified minimum standards for treatment and mandated independent monitoring of the state's response. In 1977, in *Halderman v. Pennhurst State School and Hospital et al.,* the very existence of state institutions was challenged. In Minnesota's *Welsch v. Likens* (1974), the federal District Court Consent Decree stipulated the types of staff required to be employed and the levels of staff supervision the state was required to meet.

Services Provided by Other Units of Government

In the 1980s, services provided by other units of government emphasized case management that formalized the county social services' role in coordinating and directing the clients' interdisciplinary teams. This change increased and formalized the county's presence in facilitating care for its citizens with developmental disabilities and made the county, state, and federal government (through Medicaid funding) partners in supporting community care. For example, in Minnesota, state services are considered the "safety net" for a limited number of court-committed individuals with severely challenging behaviors who pose a threat to public safety. In many locales, a main consumer of crisis services is the county case manager who makes the referrals for services and receives the assessment and treatment recommendations report. Typically, county case managers also coordinate the funding for the services. The county case manager is the designated leader of the client's interdisciplinary treatment team. His or her depth of knowledge and level of assertiveness can have a profound effect on the care the client receives.

Legislation

The disabilities community, especially parents and self-advocates, has brought about many dramatic and visible improvements in care over the course of the past 50 years (ARC, 1998). Stories from that community have supplied the individual faces and the person-specific details that make funding requests urgent and believable to state legislators and members of the news media. Once society united around the desire for community integration, full inclusion became a highly valued and necessary pursuit. Parents' and care-providers' testimonies advocating the need for crisis prevention and response services were a key reason for their development.

The belief in community integration was recently strengthened by the United States Supreme Court decision in *Olmstead v. L. C. et al.* (1999). According to the

Healthcare Finance Administration's letter to state Medicare directors (Westmoreland & Perez, 2000), a case was brought by two Georgia women whose disabilities included mental retardation and mental illness. They resided in state-operated institutions even though their interdisciplinary team believed they could be served in community-based treatment programs. Plaintiffs' attorneys asserted that continued institutionalization was a violation of their rights under the Americans With Disabilities Act (ADA; 1990). The Court found that Title II of the ADA obligated the state to provide treatment services in the most appropriate integrated setting. The unjustified isolation was found to be based on disability. Thus, the ADA, as interpreted in light of the *Olmstead* decision, requires states to avoid discrimination on the basis of disability by serving clients in the most integrated settings appropriate to their needs. The Court indicated the state may meet its obligation by developing comprehensive, effectively working plans for placing clients in the most integrated setting appropriate.

Current Services by Existing Practitioners

In some locations supportive services existed with community-based vendors operating prior to the development of crisis prevention and response services. For example, a small number of psychologists and psychiatrists provided behavioral consultation to treatment teams serving Medicaid-eligible clients. Intellectual testing, diagnostic assessment, and limited consultation with the individual's treatment team were services reimbursable through Medicaid. Individual and group psychotherapy were also provided for higher-functioning clients (i.e., generally those with moderate or mild intellectual deficits). Most of the necessary assessments and treatment were provided either at the client's residence or day treatment and habilitation program. Psychiatric care was a more difficult service to access. Providers of other therapies (e.g., occupational, speech, and physical therapy) also were available prior to the development of crisis response and prevention services, but specialized behavioral consultation remained a difficult-to-obtain specialty.

Advocacy Effects

The development of crisis prevention and response services is of great interest to the advocacy community, supporting the benefits of community integration and replacing or reducing the frequency of emergency psychiatric hospitalizations. Those who need crisis services are a very small percentage of the entire population of citizens with developmental disabilities.

Trade Union Agreements

In many states employees of state-operated services are unionized and have collective bargaining agreements. Privately employed workers in crisis services generally do not have these arrangements. With the accelerated closure of the state-operated institutions, the development of crisis services became an attractive option to employee unions. The unions supported the development of smaller state-residential programs and state-operated day treatment and habilitation programs, as well as state-operated crisis response teams. This growth in state-operated crisis services helped maintain union jobs, and it provided continuity of care for former state hospital residents, especially those clients who chronically exhibited challenging behaviors and proved difficult to place in community sites.

Characteristics of Clients Served in Crisis Services Programs

Here we turn to the characteristics and needs of the people who have used crisis prevention and response services. Some of the primary defining characteristics are the prevalence of challenging behaviors that include aggression toward others, self-injury, property destruction, and concurrent mental illness manifestations.

Many clients served in crisis services are children and adolescents who are dually diagnosed with a mental health disorder and a developmental disability. For example, two of the many good sources of information about these dually diagnosed individuals are the *Mental Health Aspects of Developmental Disabilities*[1] and the National Association for the Dually Diagnosed (NADD), with their journal, the *NADD Bulletin*.[2] Individuals with mental heath disorders often exhibit symptom-specific challenging behaviors frequently characterized by their diagnosis (American Psychiatric Association, DSM-IV, 1994). Care providers need to be skillful in preventing the clients from displaying behaviors resulting in serious injury to themselves or others.

Individuals with mental health problems, in addition to their developmental disability, are frequently difficult to serve because they can "fall between the cracks" of services in the healthcare system. It is usually organized to serve the individuals with mental illness who have average intellectual abilities or, alternatively, developmental disabled individuals who are well adjusted and do not evidence an emotional or mental disturbance. The ages of people served in crisis programs can vary from young children to senior citizens. Because of the concurrent mental illness often observed in this population, the years from adolescence to early adulthood are often critical. Males due to their greater size and strength often exhibit more potentially dangerous challenging behaviors than do females.

---

[1] Available from Psych-Media, Inc., P.O. Box 57, Bear Creek, NC 27207-0057.
[2] Available from NADD, 132 Fair St., Kingston, NY 12401-4802.

Service Needs of Crisis Services Recipients

Crisis services recipients, especially those with mental health disorders and developmental disabilities, often require psychotropic medication in addition to positive behavioral support programs to manage their behavior and mental illness symptoms. It is noteworthy that in the past 10 years, very effective medications, specifically the atypical antipsychotics (e.g., Clozaril [clozapine], Risperdal [risperidone], Zyprexa [olanzapine], Seroquel [quetiapine], and Geodon [ziprasidone]), have been released as well as the selective serotonin reuptake inhibitor antidepressants (Prozac [fluoxetine], Zoloft [sertraline], Paxil [paroxetine], Luvox [fluvaxamine], and Celexa [citalopram]). Their use has greatly reduced potential side effects and has been very effective in managing challenging behaviors as well as treating psychosis, depression, and irritability (Kern, 1999; chap. 12, this volume).

Supervision
Generally, with this dually diagnosed population, vigilant care-provider supervision is necessary to ensure that clients do not place themselves or others at risk. Funding for residential sites where this supervision is available is often provided through the Medicaid waiver authority or through the intermediate care facilities for people with mental retardation (ICF-MR). These categories of residential homes are generally staffed around the clock, 365 days a year. When a reduction in this level of supervision is deemed appropriate, supervised living facilities are usually licensed through county-licensed foster care.

Structure
Often a broad proactive approach to managing the client's challenging behaviors is accomplished by increasing the "structure" provided through the daily scheduling of activities and tasks. This also entails the contingent management of behavior using positive behavioral supports to reward independence and prosocial alternative responses to challenging behaviors. An example of this structure building is creating a schedule of 15-minute increments allotting for activities in which the client will be involved during the day and evening hours until bedtime. The events may change daily, but the general schedule should be consistent from day to day.

Consistency in Staff Expectation and Response
It is most therapeutic when care providers follow specific training approaches with the client and respond to his or her challenging behavior in a deliberate and systematic manner. This is often referred to by the treating staff as the "consistency of program implementation." Without staff consistency, there will be varied staff response to the client's positive or challenging behaviors and differing expectations

concerning his or her level of independence. This creates a more difficult learning environment for the client. Inconsistent response by care providers is often a setting event for challenging behaviors and can make the crisis situation even more problematic. To achieve consistency, crisis staff must work diligently to increase communication among the care providers. Explicitly detailed, written treatment plans are also helpful, allowing care providers to deliver similar rewards and instructional consequences across settings. In some states, the county case manager has the responsibility for facilitating this comprehensive consistency of care among the various service-providing agencies.

The fluctuating American economy has made the challenge of consistent staff response more difficult. The many employment opportunities available to potential job applicants result in positions remaining unfilled. Consequently, workers' shifts are sometimes filled by staff from temporary agencies. These staff members are often not experienced in providing behavioral interventions.

The robust economy has also resulted in greater staff turnover with direct care staff moving among agencies or leaving the field for new opportunities. Frequent staff changes create a great challenge in ensuring staff consistency in responding to the client's behavior. Reliable and consistent staffing remain very problematic.

System Planning

When developing crisis services, system planning needs to ensure that services will be comprehensive and coordinated. Often this begins with the counties developing services individually or collaborating with neighboring counties on a regional basis. Rural counties may form regional cooperative agencies to develop and oversee crisis services. State agencies are often involved due to the funding and regulatory requirements. State employees who had extensive previous experience with the clients prior to their leaving the institutions and then assisted with crisis services in the community are another component of state involvement. Similar private sector involvement occurs through formal contracts between the regional or county authorities.

An important design feature for crisis prevention and response is outpatient services at the clients' home and workplace. Thus, in practice, behavior analysts and nurses travel to where the client's behaviors actually occur. Crisis workers visit the residence, day treatment and habilitation program, or school setting to observe the interaction between care providers and the client. This naturalistic observation is dissimilar to the traditional counselor-client psychotherapeutic approach that is predominantly office-based. This orientation requires the crisis service worker to be mobile with reliable transportation and the capability of attending two, three, or four different meetings each work day. Anticipation of transportation needs and costs for the mobile workforce must be considered during the development of crisis service planning. In some cases, crisis workers have been provided cars, or they use their own vehicles and are reimbursed for mileage. When portable computers with printers are available, crisis workers can then generate their treatment reports very quickly. This ensures responsiveness and provides the referring agency with timely assistance.

Knowledgeable behavior analysts are necessary; especially those who have the maturity and experience to advise a diverse range of care providers. Ideally, this calls for a graduate-level behavior analyst who has at least a couple of years of experience in program development at either residential or day treatment and habilitation programs. Crisis workers need to be credible to family members and the staff of agencies. Good writing skills are necessary to produce timely and coherent reports, which outline the suggested treatment recommendations. An extensive knowledge of mental health and developmental disabilities resources in their service regions is also very helpful.

Consultant psychologists and psychiatrists are also important for advising the behavior analysts and psychiatric nurses on a case-by-case basis. The psychologist brings skills in intellectual and behavioral assessments as well as understanding the dynamics of the living and working situations. The psychiatrist can bring skill in medication management and additional insight into the physical conditions contributing to behavioral disturbances. This broad case consultation by behavior analysts, psychologists, psychiatrists, psychiatric nurses, occupational therapists, and individuals from other disciplines (e.g., speech therapy, dietetics, physical therapy, clinical pharmacy, and other related specialties) provide a broad foundation to assist the interdisciplinary team in making treatment decisions.

Consultative Role in the Provision of Crisis Planning and Response

Once the decision has been made to develop and operate crisis prevention and response services, the behavior analysts, nurses, psychologists, residential counselors, and other professionals who will be providing community-based assistance must be sufficiently trained. Any state or county employees reassigned from their previous work at large congregate care facilities must develop an alternative understanding of their role and the needs of their clients and stakeholders.

Community-based consultation demands much greater independence, self-direction, and assertiveness than does institutional practice. The forces operating are more aligned to those of private practice and independent contracting. At the onset of planning for crisis services, it is important to identify the customer for the proposed crisis prevention and response services.

Defining the Customer

In recent years identifying the customer and developing a mission statement has become a common business practice. This practice is not so common in human services. If college graduates without experience are hired to provide community-based crisis services, this practice is especially needed. Employees must view the consultative role in crisis services as a collaborative effort with colleagues and as a refinement and extension of the care provider's existing care, not as an investigation the purpose of which is to uncover neglect or malfeasance. The primary customer of crisis prevention and response is the client; other customers include the county case manager, family members, direct-care staff members of the residential and day programs, educational staff of the school program, and other community members. One crisis service program administrator characterized this desirable consultative role as "We're in this together" (W. Larson, personal communication, 1993). Crisis consultation is usually sought to help existing providers make behavioral assessments and develop a systematic plan to prevent future crisis incidents and improve the client's quality of life. As stated earlier, it is important to build upon the existing care provider's strengths, rather than to focus on uncovering a plethora of additional problems. When inexperienced crisis consultative staff are employed without sufficient training and supervision, ineffective results usually occur.

Communication Skills

Crisis service workers must have good communication skills, both oral and written. This is especially important for developing a treatment plan and generating a timely, written report detailing the treatment recommendations. Years of academic preparation can enhance communication skills. The crisis service worker should independently produce the written report. This task is highly demanding and necessary for responsive consultation.

Analytical Reasoning

Crisis service workers should be able to fully understand the client's social and physical environment. It is especially useful to have an understanding of the underlying agency or interdisciplinary team conflicts. When crisis services are initiated, technical assistance in behavior analysis or psychopharmacotherapy may be seen as the primary unmet need. But as additional information is gathered, it may become evident that the major problem is an uncooperative relationship within the treatment team. Such factors include divorced or divorcing parents; advocating siblings; residential programs with feuding shifts of workers; day programs in conflict with residential programs; unresponsive school districts; physicians, psychologists, and nurses who are philosophically opposed to treatment modalities; and county and state representatives who are unable or unwilling to submit requests for additional funding. Often these underlying problems have not been adequately addressed and clients' challenging behavior may intensify due to the unresolved conflicts. A recipe for disaster and failure is ill-prepared crisis service workers attempting to remedy these unresolved, often long-standing, disputes.

We suggest that experienced psychologists and psychiatrists be available to discuss these situations and the possible dynamics. This consultation builds the confidence of the crisis workers in understanding the clients' diverse situations and proposing practical treatment recommendations. This type of wisdom is usually gained only through experience.

The referral from the county case manager for crisis services is often for a "second opinion" to assist the team in resolving a conflict among team participants. Bringing in an outside consultant without a previous history with the case can provide a fresh appraisal of the situation and facilitate consensus among the interdisciplinary team members concerning the direction of future treatment. Often when behavioral interventions are recommended, the care providers will respond that this is what they have already attempted and abandoned because it was ineffective or only partially effective. The crisis worker's challenge is to encourage the care provider to implement the redesigned procedures in a more consistent and precise manner. Subtle changes in the reinforcement contingencies, setting events, antecedents, or the instructional situation can produce profound changes in the client's behavior. The challenge for the crisis workers when recommending treatment strategies is to present each as an option for the team to consider the "contextual fit" (Albin, Lucyshyn, Horner, & Flannery, 1996). In most instances, the recommendations are refinements of what has already occurred or been previously considered. Here, the crisis worker's contribution is to recognize and build upon the work that has already occurred. Often it involves encouragement to be more systematic, facilitate referrals to additional expert resources, and enhance communication among the interdisciplinary team members.

Challenges of Temporary Residential Treatment

One primary challenge of offering temporary residential treatment as a crisis intervention is to have and maintain time-limited client lengths-of-stay necessary to ensure bed availability. Pressures commonly exist to exceed the predetermined maximum lengths-of-stay. It is important to anticipate these pressures when designing services and to confirm the "cannot exceed" nature of the maximum allowable length-of-stay in all discussions with family members, care providers, and county case managers. Past experience has reliably demonstrated the average length-of-stay tends to fall in the 80th to 100th percentile of the maximum allowable length-of-stay.

Another difficult challenge involves the recruitment of skilled staff for the temporary residential program. Because of the concurrent mental illness that many of the admitted crisis clients experience, personnel with previous experience in mental health settings, in addition to experience in developmental disabilities, can be very helpful. A high staff-client ratio (e.g., 1 staff for 2 clients) can greatly facilitate treatment. An hourly pay differential has worked to encourage veteran employees to transfer into crisis services from other work settings.

Inexperienced staff often draw erroneous conclusions when observing the bizarre maladaptive behavior of a client with mental illness and mental retardation. A false belief is frequently expressed that a client is voluntarily choosing to act in an irrational and disturbed manner. This speculation concerning the client's behavior assumes his or her motivation is generally to irritate staff. These false assumptions support the resulting erroneous conclusion that it is necessary to be strict and punitive when correcting the client's aberrant behavior. The crisis worker's emphasis has to be positively oriented to ensure enduring treatment gains. The staff member who is the most outspoken about the client's problematic behavior often is the most dissatisfied about their agency's slow response addressing the "crisis." These staff members frequently perceive themselves as victims of the client's aberrant behavior.

When providing temporary residential crisis treatment, avoid focusing exclusively on the residential side of the crisis services. With sufficient resources, the client's behavior will improve while in temporary residential treatment. The greater challenge is actively planning and facilitating the treatment gains to generalize to the previous community-based settings. The community outreach side of crisis prevention and response, whenever possible, can provide the most enduring and cost-effective gains. Temporary residential treatment becomes necessary only when in-home treatment is ineffective after a protracted intervention period.

The term *crisis services* in developmental disabilities often is a misnomer for behavioral consultation and treatment recommendations or proactive intervention strategies. Very rarely will a behavior analyst, nurse, psychologist, or others be needed immediately to drive to the client's care setting to intervene in a chaotic and possibly life-threatening situation similar to those experienced in the mental health field.

When crisis services were initially developed, a perceived service need was immediate responsiveness to de-escalate a disturbed client's behavior. This perceived service was unrealistic because the dangerous behavior generally de-escalated before the arrival of the crisis worker while the actual function of these staff workers was behavioral consultation. Crisis services are proactive, not reactive, and build on the skills of the existing care providers to assist in preventing institutionalization and enhancing the positive lifestyle of the clients served.

Summary

This chapter has described seven forces (litigation, existing services provided by other units of governments, legislation responding to wishes of family members and care providers, current services by existing providers, advocacy effects, trade union agreements, and the desire to spend Medicaid more wisely) that influence the development and provision of crisis services. In addition, the characteristics of the clients served in crisis services programs were discussed, as were the needs of the recipients — the enhanced need for supervision, structure, and consistency in staff expectations and responses.

Suggestions were made for system planning, including the consultative role in the provision of crisis planning and response, the need to define the customer and consumer of crisis services, and the desirable skills in communication and analytic reasoning for crisis service workers.

Challenges of providing temporary residential treatment and of describing crisis services were likewise considered.

The systematic and comprehensive provision of crisis prevention and response services helps clients with developmental disabilities and severe challenging behavior, many times coupled with mental health disorders, remain in the community, enhancing their independence and self-determination.

Author Note

The views expressed are those of the authors and do not represent those of the Minnesota Department of Human Services or any of its agencies. The authors thank Jane Moore Clark for her review and suggestions.

References

Albin, R. W., Lucyshyn, J. M., Horner, R. H., & Flannery, K. B. (1996). Contextual fit for behavioral support plans: A model for "Goodness of Fit." In L. K. Koegel, R. L. Koegel, & G. Dunlap (Eds.), *Positive behavioral support: Including people with difficult behavior in the community* (pp. 81–98). Baltimore: Paul H. Brookes.

American Psychiatric Association. (1994). *Diagnostic and statistical manual of mental disorders* (4th ed.). Washington, DC: Author.

Americans With Disabilities Act of 1990, 42 U.S.C.A. § 12101 *et seq.* (West 1993).

ARC. (1998). *Visions and victories: Celebrating 50 years of creating opportunities.* Minneapolis: ARC of Hennepin County.

Chafee, J. H. (1988, March 22). Opening statement of Hon. John H. Chafee. In G. Mitchell (Chair), Hearing before the Subcommittee on Health on the Medicaid Home and Community Quality Services Act of 1987 (S. Hrg. 100-817, pp. 2–5). Washington, DC: U.S. Government Printing Office.

Halderman v. Pennhurst State School and Hospital, 466 F. Supp. 1295 (U.S. Third Circuit Court of Appeals, 1978).

Kern, C. A. (1999). Psychopharmacotherapy for people with profound and severe mental retardation and mental disorders. In N. A. Wieseler & R. H. Hanson (Eds.), *Challenging behavior of persons with mental health disorders and severe developmental disabilities* (pp.103–112). Washington, DC: American Association on Mental Retardation.

Olmstead v. L.C., 527 U.S. 581.596 (1999).

Scheerenberger, R. C. (1983). *A history of mental retardation.* Baltimore: Paul H. Brookes.

Welsch v. Likins, 373 F. Supp. 487 (D. Minn., 1974).

Westmoreland, T. M., & Perez, T. (2000). *Guidance on Olmstead decision and fact sheet.* Baltimore: Health Care Financing Administration.

Wyatt v. Stickney, 344 F. Supp. 373 (M.D. Alabama, 1972).

PART 2

State and Regional Networks of Behavioral Support and Crisis Response

CHAPTER 3

The Vermont Crisis Intervention Network: Nine Years of Prevention

Patrick Frawley
Elia Vecchione
Vermont Crisis Intervention Network
Moretown, Vermont

With the national movement toward deinstitutionalization, community-based crisis services for people with developmental disabilities (DD) have become increasingly essential. Although some very good programs are currently in operation, there is a paucity of professional literature regarding the efficacy of such programs. This chapter describes the development, implementation and outcomes achieved by the Vermont Crisis Intervention Network (VCIN), a statewide crisis prevention and intervention program, which originated in March 1991.

It is vitally important for readers to understand the context in which this program operates. Vermont is a small and rural state with a population of just over 600,000. Approximately one quarter of these people live in Chittenden County, which includes the small city of Burlington. Vermont is 157 miles long and only 90 miles at its widest point along the border with Canada. The state narrows dramatically as one travels south. This combination of population and geography allows for easy statewide communication and cooperation. For instance, it is not difficult to gather all of the directors of developmental disabilities programs for a meeting on a regular basis. And when all of these people are together, there are only about 15 of them in the room. In many states the population and geography of Vermont equate to a county or a region.

Vermont's current service system for people with developmental disabilities is also worth describing in some detail, to provide further information on the context in which VCIN functions. There are nine full-service community mental health centers with programs for people with developmental disabilities. Beyond these agencies there are six smaller agencies that provide only DD services. These agencies together currently serve an estimated 2,400 consumers (Vermont Division of Developmental Services, 2000). Residential services within all of the above-mentioned agencies are based primarily upon a shared-living model. Within this arrangement individuals with DD live in the homes of people who provide them with care. Obviously, the level of care varies by individual. This reliance upon individualized residential care is an important and unique aspect to Vermont's service system. It will be important to remember these contextual issues as this chapter unfolds.

History

Vermont has had a long history of reliance upon institutions to provide care for people with DD. Opened in 1915, the Brandon Training School (BTS) was the only major institution in Vermont specifically housing people. In addition, for years some people with DD and psychiatric disorders or very challenging behavior lived at the Vermont State Hospital (VSH). Slowly, through the 1970s, 1980s, and into the early 1990s, the census of these institutions was decreased through community placement. In 1991 the decision was made to close BTS and move to a completely community-based system for people with DD. In addition to this closure, it was decided that access to VSH for people with DD would be dramatically restricted. Two years prior to the announced closure of BTS, we (authors) proposed VCIN to Vermont state officials. The impetus for this program was our experience providing clinical consultation throughout Vermont through the end of the 1980s. In March 1991, with the BTS closure determined, state officials gave their approval, created a funding mechanism, and VCIN was launched. In late 1993 the last person moved from BTS and Vermont's entirely community-based system was in operation.

Vermont Crisis Intervention Network

VCIN's primary function is to prevent the institutionalization of any Vermont resident with developmental disabilities. Beyond this goal the program strives to enhance the clinical services provided to these individuals through the service system in Vermont. This is attempted through a three-tiered service approach. Within the first level, prevention-oriented services are provided. At Level 2 early intervention efforts are evident, and at Level 3 short-term community-based, crisis residential services are used. These aspects of the program are further described below. VCIN serves a vital role in the maintenance of the stability of the community system. This role, though, is one played in collaboration with all of the agencies serving individuals with DD in Vermont. It would be completely erroneous to assume that the success of the program is due to our staff only. Without the intense dedication of the community agencies to serve every person with DD within the community, VCIN would not be successful.

Staffing

The program is staffed as follows: Patrick Frawley, with a PhD in psychology, as full-time director. Elia Vecchione, with the same credentials, provides consultation services to the program 1 to 2 days per week and coordinates the Level 3 services. Our staff includes a psychiatrist and a nurse for 1 day per week. Additionally, there are three full-time and one part-time direct service staff who work primarily within Level 3 (see below).

Level 1: The Clinical Network

There are not enough highly trained clinicians practicing in Vermont to cover all of the agencies serving people with developmental disabilities. Therefore, to reduce, and potentially prevent, crises throughout the state, the level of clinical expertise within the agencies must be increased.

This founding premise was true in 1991 when VCIN was started, and it is certainly still true 9 years later. There are only a handful of clinicians in Vermont who are capable of providing sophisticated clinical consultation concerning the challenging behavior and dual diagnosis issues presented by people with DD. The prevention of crises, and especially the need for the relocation of a person with DD from his or her home, can be dramatically reduced through the increasing of clinical competencies of the agency staff. A clear primary prevention orientation is evident within Level 1. This is accomplished through a number of activities.

The primary service within Level 1 (see Table 3.1) is the monthly network meeting, which gathers the primary clinical staff from each agency. Most often the staff who attend are experienced case-manager-level employees. In addition to agency staff, the Vermont Division of Developmental Services is always represented. Other interested participants are always welcome as well.

Within these meetings we deliver training on any number of topics ranging from identifying dual diagnosis to the need for psychotherapy to treatment of self-injurious behavior. These trainings are provided by the Network staff or by experts from outside the Network. Also at the monthly meetings, we have agency staff present challenging clinical situations in which they are involved. These presentations serve a number of functions. First, they allow for the presenting staff to re-

---

TABLE 3.1
Vermont Crisis Intervention Network Program Components

Level 1: The Clinical Network
    Prevention Orientation
        Monthly meetings
            Trainings
            Individual situation presentations
        State-wide trainings

Level 2: On-Site Consultation
    Early Intervention
        Psychological
        Psychiatric

Level 3: Crisis Residential Services
    Safe, Humane, Clinically Sophisticated Residential Care
        Stabilization
        Evaluation

---

ceive support and suggestions regarding the stressful situation. Second, other meeting participants observe models of problem analysis and generation of potential solutions. In this way, each meeting participant is further trained in clinical assessment and treatment. Third, the Level 1 meeting provides a true "network" of professionals who know, and one hopes, come to trust one another. This meeting has proven to be quite valuable as very challenging behavior arises within this community system. For the entire system to function well, it has been, and will continue to be, important that community agencies rely on each other for support and cooperation.

Other functions of Level 1 include trainings, which may take place at a community agency or may involve specifically selected participants. For instance, a few years ago we had identified that many psychiatrists in Vermont who were seeing patients with DD were not especially skilled in their abilities to diagnose and treat people with such needs. In an effort to increase the competencies of these psychiatrists, we arranged a conference with a well-known and well-respected psychiatrist who specializes in the treatment of individuals with DD. We invited only psychiatrists and had a good turnout. This is in complete accordance with Level 1 goals of increasing the clinical abilities of those who work with our population in an effort to reduce or prevent crises. We have planned for years to provide a similar conference for providers of psychotherapy, as finding competent and willing therapists is an ongoing concern.

Level 2: On-Site Consultation

To reduce or prevent crises, expert clinical services can be delivered within the local agencies. Stabilization of a potential crisis is often realized through early intervention. Clinical staff, direct service staff, and case manager competencies can be increased through this consultation.

Within Level 2, expert clinical services are provided to agency staff at their location and in reference to a specific individual. Most of the Level 2 activity involves psychological or psychiatric consultation to teams addressing the issues of challenging behavior or dual diagnosis. This is clearly an early intervention strategy.

Level 2 consultation through the Network involves a flexible but fairly consistent format. A referral may come from anywhere, state personnel, agency staff, parents, and so forth. The primary consideration is that the individuals being referred must qualify for developmental services within Vermont. It is not necessary that they are served by an agency within the Network, or that they receive any services at all. Following a determination of eligibility, one of the authors (Frawley or Vecchione) makes an initial contact, evaluating the services desired and determining which VCIN personnel are most appropriate for the consultation. Depending on the demands of the consultation, one or more of the professional staff may become involved. Some consultations require both psychological and psychiatric expertise, but often the request is for one or the other. There are subtle differences to the consultations of each discipline, and they presented in detail below.

Psychological Consultation

As is true in Level 1, raising the competencies of local staff (direct service staff as well as case managers) is among the primary interests of our consultants at Level 2. We strive to inform and educate as well as support through our consultations. This is a bit more challenging at Level 2, where the dynamics at play seem to try to force us into an expert role, dictating plans to staff. Yet it is important that when the consultation is completed, the staff has learned new skills and has had confidence raised in its own abilities to solve clinical issues. We hope this is accomplished through our consultation format, which is quite straightforward. A fully detailed description of our consultation approach is beyond the scope of this chapter, but a cursory description, touching on the high points, is provided.

The first task of the consultant at Level 2 is to convince the local agency staff that the consultant is not a threat. There is often a good deal of resistance to the "expert" consultant, who can be perceived as an overeducated know-it-all who has never really worked for a living. This situation is best overcome through honest investigation into the situation. In the process of collecting information about the consumer and his or her problem behavior, the staff (or parents, caregivers, etc.) can easily be convinced, and rightly so, that they are the ones who know this person best and that their opinions and ideas about what is going on with the person are very important. Relationships can be damaged just as easily by the consultant feeling that he or she must figure out the solution to the problem and that the staff are merely informants to his or her genius.

After collecting some introductory information from staff or case managers, we always spend a good deal of time reading the records of the consumer we are there to assist. Essential information about the history of the problem behavior is often contained in the record. This includes medical issues, medication histories, behavioral treatment histories, and psychotherapy notes.

After all of the information seems to have been collected by the consultant, we convene a team meeting to discuss the situation. These meetings include direct staff, home providers, case managers, and parents and/or guardians. In these meetings an understanding of the situation is agreed upon by the participants and a plan is developed. Many times this phase of the process requires that the participants read a good deal of information about the problem behavior and potential solutions. We often have direct service staff, parents, and case managers reading very technical, clinical articles during this portion of the consultation. This facilitation of their understanding is directly in line with Level 1 and 2 objectives.

It is important that the plan be designed and agreed upon by those who must carry it out. Even though there is often a great push to have the consultant devise and write the plan, a plan developed by a consultant is almost always doomed to failure. The people who have to implement the plan must be invested in it, and this is best accomplished by their designing and writing it, with assistance as needed.

After the plan is developed and implemented, we have ongoing meetings to discuss problems, successes, and modification to the plan. Depending on the situation, our consultants may follow a team for as long as a year, or may be done after a meeting or two. Table 3.2 shows the number of Level 2 consultations provided by year.

Psychiatric Consultation

Consultation of a psychiatric nature is quite similar to the above-described psychological consultation, in that consultation attempts to raise local competencies. Although it is not necessary that the staff develop the psychiatric plan, especially when it includes medication, it is essential that they understand the plan, target symptoms, expected medication effects, and potential side effects. It is uncom-

TABLE 3.2
**Vermont Crisis Intervention Network,
Level 2: People Served by Year**

Year	N
1991	40
1992	45
1993	44
1994	42
1995	50
1996	40
1997	52
1998	61
1999	63

mon for the VCIN psychiatrist to prescribe for a consumer following a consultation. The most likely scenario is that our psychiatrist would conduct an evaluation and then provide consultation to the agency or local psychiatrist or physician. This process is likely to assure appropriate treatment as well as raise the competencies of the local physician or psychiatrist when it comes to working with individuals with DD.

Level 3: Residential Crisis Services

At times, for a variety of potential reasons, it will be necessary for an individual to leave his or her home. For a full community system to operate properly, it is essential to have an alternative setting, offering safe housing, evaluation, and treatment.

Throughout the 9 years of the VCIN program, we have had a steadily decreasing number of residential crisis options. In the first year of the program, we operated two well-staffed, full-service crisis beds, and we also offered four respite options, which could accommodate individuals with less-acute demands. These options steadily decreased until we were left operating just one bed in the summer of 1995. These decreases of VCIN resources were a direct result of the increased crisis capacities within the community agencies. We have continued to operate one bed since that time and this is the service described below.

Located on a dirt road in the country, our crisis bed is a two-bedroom, two-story home, to which we have attached our offices. These spaces are separated by a large meeting room. The house has 12 acres of fields surrounding it with a small river running nearby. One of the most obvious features of the house and the surrounding grounds is that it is very quiet and serene. It is about one half mile from the center of a small town. Another feature is that it is quite safe. While retaining its "homey" feel, the house has been modified to be a safe environment for anyone who may stay with us. For instance, all of the windows are made of Plexiglas, which reduces the likelihood of injury should someone attempt to break a window.

Only one consumer at a time resides there. We have stood by this guiding premise for the duration of our program. Even though there has at times been pressure for us to allow two individuals to receive treatment there at the same time, we have not budged. We strongly believe that in order to best assist each person who comes along, we need to assure that the environment in which he or she resides is as stable, safe, and calming as possible. In this way we are most clinically effective and efficient.

Our house is staffed 24 hours per day by one VCIN staff person at a time. Approximately 3.5 full-time-equivalent staff members are required to operate this bed in a rotating shift pattern. While a person stays at this residence, he or she is provided with as meaningful a day schedule as possible. Some individuals are looking to spend some productive time working on small tasks or odd jobs; others are content to relax and take it easy. While residing in our crisis house, an individual also receives the clinical services described in Level 2. These include psychological and psychiatric evaluations and treatment. Brief supportive psychotherapy is available when appropriate as is monitoring and modification of any medications. To facilitate the continuance of any clinical or programmatic approaches instituted during a person's stay with us, Level 2 consultation services are almost always provided in a follow-up fashion once a person leaves our bed. These types of after-care services are essential to assure proper long-term implementation.

As indicated above, a variety of issues may precipitate a stay in our crisis bed. Many times an admission is due to behavioral difficulties within the consumer's home in the community. Another common precipitant is homelessness. Furthermore, some individuals stay with us to receive a close-up evaluation of their behavior. Access to the bed is controlled by personnel at the Vermont Division of Developmental Services (VTDDS), which allows the VCIN program to maintain a pleasant neutrality when it comes to deciding who can stay and for how long.

While a person is residing in our crisis bed, there are a number of specific requirements to which the sending agency (if there is one) must adhere. First and foremost, the sending agency retains its role as case manager, continuing to be responsible for all of the regular services it usually provides (e.g., medical coordination, Medicaid issues of any sort, etc.). Beyond this, the agency is responsible to attend a weekly clinical meeting regarding the person residing within the bed. This meeting is attended by all VCIN staff, a representative from VTDDS, the consumer's guardian (if one exists), and staff from the sending agency empowered to make clinical, residential, and financial decisions. This decision-making power is essential for the meetings to be efficient and productive. At this meeting decisions are made concerning treatment approaches, medication changes, and plans for return to the sending agency, including target discharge dates. The program tries to stick to a 30-day limit, although this is certainly flexible depending on the situation.

Throughout the life of the project, there has been an increase in the efficiency of the entire system, not only to avoid crises in general, but to accelerate the return of displaced individuals. In our first few years of operation, many people stayed for a great length of time. The record stay is 216 days, and at the same time another person stayed for 206 days. Clearly, the residential portion of the crisis service was not being effective during these times. Directly following these lengthy stays, a new understanding of crisis-bed utilization was developed by a committee of Network and agency representatives. This group advised that for the entire state crisis system to be effective, a person staying in the VCIN bed could not always stay there until the optimal residential situation was located. There would be times when a person would have to leave the bed and transition to a situation that was safe but not perfect. In the past we had been waiting until a very solid residential program could be designed. This policy had a direct and rapid effect on our service. We became an extremely efficient group when it came to assessing a person and assisting that person in moving on. This did result in some people perceiving the crisis bed as simply a place to stay for a short time versus somewhere to go for a meaningful and possibly prolonged treatment. Yet this streamlining was essential, especially when VCIN was reduced to the current one-bed status.

Table 3.3 reveals the use of Level 3 from the inception of the program through the end of 1999. These data show how our beds have been used, indicating how many people were served and the average length of stay. Clearly, since 1995, when we reduced our service to one crisis bed, we have been very efficient in assisting individuals to move on from our service. A great number of the individuals served at this level were certainly diverted from institutional placements, although an exact calculation of these diversions is not possible. For fiscal year 1999, according to the Vermont Division of Developmental Services *Annual Report* (2000), only two people with DD spent any time within the Vermont State (psychiatric) Hospital. Additionally, the report indicates that the VCIN bed was full during both of these individuals' stays within the hospital. Had our bed been open, they would have, most likely, been served within our crisis bed. Obviously, this is reflective of a very efficient statewide service system.

We feel we offer people who are in crisis a safe, humane, and clinically sophisticated environment in which they can become stabilized, receive evaluation, and/or simply take it easy before returning to their lives within the community.

TABLE 3.3
Vermont Crisis Intervention Network,
Level 3: People Served per Year

Year	N	Total Days	M Stay (Days)
1991	15	480	32.0
1992	20	605	30.2
1993	15	816	54.4
1994	11	578	52.5
1995	13	211	16.2
1996	15	219	14.6
1997	10	274	27.4
1998	13	271	20.9
1999	12	255	21.3
Total	124	3,709	29.9

Note: Program reduced to one crisis bed in 1995.

Case Examples

To facilitate a further understanding of the intricate functioning of our program with the Vermont service system, we present two in-depth discussions of actual clinical services delivered. These situations were chosen as representative of our program's interactions with other agencies.

Level 2: "Dave"

A case manager from an agency within our state called our program to request a psychiatric or psychological evaluation. The case manager described over the phone how a young man named Dave (age 23), to whom they had provided services for a number of years, had somewhat suddenly stopped attending his vocational and recreational activities and was eating dramatically less. He had begun to communicate less with those around him. In fact, it seemed to people that Dave was losing all kinds of skills he had previously displayed. In addition, he was spending almost all of his time in his bedroom and would not interact with people when they entered his room to speak with him. Of great concern to his family, Dave was experiencing something his family referred to as "spells." During these periods he became totally enraged and stormed around the house. It was not clear to anyone what these incidents were about, although some people who had witnessed these episodes said it appeared he was speaking with people who were not present. The agency psychiatrist had some ideas about what might be at work in this situation but was uncertain about how to proceed and desired some assistance in diagnosis and treatment options.

Through this telephone interview, it appeared to our program staff that there was a high probability that some sort of psychiatric disorder was evidenced by this young man. Because of this our psychiatrist was the first of our consultants to be involved with this man's team. She conducted her standard psychiatric evaluation and determined, in her opinion, that Dave was showing signs of a major depression. She contacted the agency psychiatrist and discussed some treatment options. They met together with the clinical team and Dave's family and decided to proceed with a trial of an antidepressant.

Over the course of 3 months, Dave's behavior improved. He was having fewer behavioral outbursts, his eating had returned to normal, he was communicating more with those around him, and he was coming out of his bedroom more. All of this was fantastic, but he still was not able to leave his home and reengage in his life. He still spent long hours in his room and appeared, at times, to be unable to enjoy the company of others. Interestingly, he would leave the home only to help his mother bring in groceries from her car, a distance of about 20 feet from his front door.

At this time the case manager called our program again to ask if we could help them think about what might be going on with Dave. Through discussion among our program's professional staff, we decided we would send one of our psychology consultants to look into the situation and attempt to assist Dave, his family, and the agency staff.

Conducting our standard psychological consultation, our staff person reviewed Dave's records and interviewed staff and the family. He also spent some time with Dave at his home. Our staff found him to be free of dramatic symptoms of depression but evidencing what appeared to be agoraphobia. It appeared his symptoms of depression were lifted by the antidepressant, but he was still left with some anxiety about reentering the world. In discussions with Dave's team, it was decided that a standard desensitization program would be conducted by the agency staff. The plan was for the staff to first attempt to interact with Dave in his bedroom, to build a relationship. He responded well to this, and through some subtle encouragement, he and a staff person slowly moved their relationship to the kitchen. This slow transition was fraught with setbacks. Dave would often retreat to his room. His team was very clear that they were not going to pressure him to stay out of his room. They acted as if they really did not care that he retreated, but would positively respond when he decided to be out of his room. This is an essential point. They felt they could not "push" but just had to offer the positive aspects of interacting with people. They also refrained from building any contingency program around this behavior, fearing the focus would heighten Dave's anxiety in general.

As he became more comfortable with the staff person, the two of them ventured out, first onto the porch a few times. Then, building on the fact that Dave was used to helping his mother with groceries, the staff person started bringing groceries. Dave was very willing to assist her. One day the staff person brought a basketball to the house. Dave had reportedly liked to shoot baskets in his driveway but hadn't for months. Instead of "pushing" the ball on him, by making a direct offer to play, the staff person "accidentally" dropped the ball out of the car onto the ground one day when they were bringing in the groceries. Dave picked up the ball and dribbled it a couple of times and then set it down. The staff member picked up the ball and bounced it to Dave. This became a routine for a day or two, then one day the staff person shot the ball at the basket and the game was on.

The staff member used a very similar technique to get Dave to ride in her car. His mother had always placed her groceries in the trunk. Of course the staff person initially copied this location for her groceries. But one day, she placed one of the grocery bags in the back seat. She slowly, over time, placed all of the groceries in the back and some in the front seat of the car. Obviously, within a few days they were going for rides and finally getting him back to his vocational and recreational activities.

During this entire desensitization phase, which lasted about two months, we had numerous team meetings to review progress and plan our next steps. We have not heard from Dave, his family, or his staff since. This is a nice example of how Level 2 (on-site consultation) works. Expert clinical services (psychiatric and psychological) are available to local agencies to access as needed. With the capability of intensive follow-along, consultations do not become one-shot, write-a-report-and-move-on situations. These folks in this example needed ongoing assistance to figure out exactly how to approach the complex psychiatric and psychological issues exhibited by this young man.

Level 3: "Dianne"

Dianne, age 15, had experienced a traumatic life filled with abuse and multiple residential placements. We became aware of her through the usual method. We were called by an agency that was having trouble meeting her needs. She was living with a very dedicated couple, struggling with some of Dianne's challenging behavior. When Dianne became upset, she became extremely violent, smashing things within the house and becoming aggressive toward her home providers.

Our consultation to Dianne and her team followed the customary route, with record review, interviews, and observations. Her main issue was that Dianne had great difficulty controlling herself when she became upset about anything. Our consultant provided extensive training to Dianne's team regarding trauma and abuse issues and attachment issues, as well as anger control. In addition, the team had decided to try to locate a therapist who could engage Dianne around some of the intense psychological issues of her past.

During the course of our consultation to this team, Dianne engaged in some very destructive and aggressive behavior that resulted in her home providers deciding that they could no longer have Dianne live with them. As is often the case, the home providers said Dianne needed to move immediately. The agency that served Dianne did not have any crisis or respite options available, so they requested a stay at the VCIN crisis bed. Since the bed was open at the time, an admission was approved by the VTDDS representative serving the role of "gate keeper."

Dianne came immediately to our house in the country, where we conducted an intake assessment. In this situation, our intake person was the same consultant who had provided consultation to Dianne and her team, so we were quite familiar with her needs.

Dianne stayed in our Level 3 service for 37 days. This was somewhat longer than is customary, but such a lengthy stay was required because the sending agency had determined that they could no longer provide services to Dianne. Finding a new provider agency and then a new home within that agency can be a somewhat lengthy process. While Dianne stayed with us, our psychiatrist prescribed changes in psychiatric medication. Our psychiatrist had taken over prescribing from the sending agency psychiatrist, because it was obvious that Dianne would no longer be served by the sending agency. While residing in our bed, Dianne also received short-term anger control treatment. She responded well to her stay in our bed, with some, but minimal, disruptive behavior noted. The staff of the crisis bed are well trained, seasoned veterans, with years of experience within our field. It also helped, in this instance, that they were all males. Dianne had a history of being able to control herself better when in the presence of men. (This is not always the case. Many times people staying with us prefer the company of women and are able to feel more comfortable and in control with them as care providers. We just happened to have all men on our staff at the time Dianne came to be with us.)

After the new agency came forward, sending representatives to meet Dianne, they searched for a new home for her. This search was fairly productive, with two potential home providers identified. Both of these new home providers spent some time with Dianne, first at our house and then at their home and, finally, in the community. Both were interested in having her live with them, but Dianne had a stronger liking for one of the homes. Dianne's guardian from Vermont Social and Rehabilitative Services agreed that the home Dianne had selected was a good choice. We began having Dianne spend more and more time at her new home, with some overnight stays included. Finally everyone was certain that things would go well and Dianne moved to her new home.

We continued to provide Level 2 follow-up services to Dianne and her new home providers. Her new case manager had trouble finding Dianne a new therapist who could continue the anger control treatments, so we offered to provide Dianne with continued treatment until a new therapist could be found. Our psychiatrist transferred Dianne's prescriptions to the psychiatrist of the new agency with an offer of continued consultation.

There were certainly many rocky moments for Dianne and her new home providers during the initial few weeks, but they all made it through these challenging times together. Dianne has been living in this home for 2 years. Our involvement now is quite minimal. We do provide some Level 2 consultation to Dianne's team as needed.

This description is fairly representative of our Level 3 service, although most stays are for a shorter duration and most people do not change agencies while staying in our service.

Summary

For 9 years the developmental disabilities service system within Vermont has collaboratively provided prevention, early intervention, and crisis residential services to its residents with developmental disabilities. The Vermont Crisis Intervention Network continues to play an important role in this service provision.

References

Vermont Division of Developmental Services. (2000). *Annual Report 2000.* Waterbury: Author.

CHAPTER 4

The Minnesota Crisis System:
A Public-Private Collaboration[1]

Norman A. Wieseler
Eastern Minnesota Community Support Services
Faribault, Minnesota

Ronald H. Hanson
Joan M. Oslund
Mount Olivet Rolling Acres
Victoria, Minnesota

Over the past 30 years, the lives of people with developmental disabilities have dramatically changed. They have moved from large congregate care facilities, many built during the asylum era, to integrated community settings where work and living skills are congruent with the prevailing societal standards of conduct. Social, political, economic, and legal influences have propelled the deinstitutionalization movement at an accelerating rate (Anderson, Lakin, Mangan, & Prouty, 1998). The magnitude of the trend has depended upon the geographic location and time period.

Since 1967 the number of institutions serving individuals with developmental disabilities has dramatically decreased. In 1967 the daily average number of individuals residing in state and psychiatric institutions reached an all-time high of 228,500. Between 1960 and 1971, only two state institutions in the United States

[1] The views expressed are those of the authors and do not represent an official endorsement by the Minnesota Department of Human Services or any of its agencies.

closed (0.17 per year); from 1972 to 1975, five institutions closed (1.25 per year). Between 1976 and 1979, five institutions were closed (1.5 per year), and from 1980 to 1987, 26 institution closings occurred (3.25 per year). From 1988 to 1991, institution closures increased to 34 (8.5 per year), and from 1992 to 1997, 67 institutions closed (11.2 per year). At present, this accelerating trend continues and will likely proceed until only small specialized facilities remain (Anderson et al., 1998).

This trend produced enhanced lifestyles for clients. This change presented new challenges for care providers and planners to make community living successful (Lakin, Hayden, & Abery, 1994). Individuals who have long-standing patterns of aggression and destructiveness are especially challenging to maintain in their community placements. Numerous studies (e.g., Intagliata & Willer, 1982; Scheerenberger, 1981; Schroeder, Rojahn, & Oldenquist, 1989) have revealed that a primary reason for unsuccessful community living and a return to an institution-like placement is the prevalence of challenging behaviors such as severe injurious attacks to oneself or others, sexual predations, and other forms of dangerous aggression or destructiveness. The community-based services required to support these at-risk individuals vary greatly from state to state (Fitzpatrick, 1995). A number of articles describing crisis prevention and response from both the state and private sectors have recently appeared (e.g., Beasley, Kroll, & Sovner, 1992; Colond & Wieseler, 1995; Davidson et al., 1995; Hanson, Oslund, & Wieseler, 1997; Jacobson & Schwartz, 1983; Pfadt & Holburn, 1996; Rudolph, Lakin, Oslund, & Larson, 1998; Sovner & DeNoyers Hurley, 1988).

Funding is critical to provide and continue community-based crisis response services to assist individuals with challenging behavior to remain in community settings and prevent transfer to more restrictive placements. For example, in Minnesota, the state legislature allocated waiver funds for both governmental and private service providers to implement community-based crisis prevention and response services. Components of these services, limited to people with mental retardation or related conditions, consist of short-term consultation to caregivers for behavioral and psychological assessment, program development, and staff training. These services are often accompanied with on-site technical assistance to provide short-term support and training in behavior analysis and intervention to prevent and respond to behavioral crises. These supports are accessed through the county case management system. As recommended by other providers of crisis prevention and intervention services (e.g., Beasley, Kroll, & Sovner, 1992; Davidson et al., 1995), the Minnesota public and private service providers receive direct funding so there is no fee for outreach services, and individuals can access these services regardless of their insurance coverage or their ability to pay. Services to people using the residential beds are financed through Medicaid or designated state and local resources.

This chapter describes the collaboration between state and private service agencies providing community-based crisis prevention and assistance in the Minneapolis-St. Paul seven-county metropolitan area of Minnesota. Although this discussion focuses on the Twin Cities, service needs throughout the state are similar. A recent survey of care providers (Nord, Wieseler, & Hanson, 1997) inquiring about the types of clients served, the support they need, and the crisis response and technical assistance necessary to prevent future behavioral crises, found broad similarities between rural and metro counties. In general, the results of this survey were consistent with the three external validity criteria described by Carr and his colleagues (Carr et al., 1999). As these authors conclude, the first need of service providers is for interventions to produce comprehensive lifestyle changes. That is, the mere reduction of the challenging behaviors jeopardizing community opportunities is not a desirable outcome unless the individual is also able to live an enhanced lifestyle commensurate to peers without behavior challenges. Second, service providers need interventions that are both practical and relevant. A competent caregiver should be able to conduct the intervention across all settings in which the person functions on a daily basis. Third, service providers need interventions to produce enduring behavioral changes. Behavior support plans lasting several years may be necessary to adequately treat clients with long-standing behavior challenges.

The development and maintenance of a comprehensive system of behavioral support to address the needs of individuals with challenging behaviors will be an emerging necessity for states undergoing deinstitutionalization. The three aforementioned external validity criteria provide guideposts in planning and implementing successful community services. It is hoped the Minnesota model of public-private collaboration will also guide the development of similar services in other states.

As stated earlier, crisis services in Minnesota are provided through a public and private collaboration. The public effort comes primarily through state employees in collaboration with the counties' social services. Eastern Minnesota Community Support Services (EMCSS) combined the "catchment areas" or regions served by the former Cambridge Human Services Center and Faribault Regional Center, both of which served only people with developmental disabilities. Private-sector crisis services are provided in two regions of Minnesota (the southeast region and Twin Cities metro area) in conjunction with the state's crisis response services.

In the Minneapolis-St. Paul metropolitan area, a seven-county area with approximately half the state's population, crisis services are coordinated through a private-sector agency, the Metro Crisis Coordination Program (MCCP). This program is overseen by a steering committee with representation from each of the seven counties. It provides outpatient consultation (preventative and emergency) and refers clients to both the public-sector EMCSS and to the private-sector Mount Olivet Rolling Acres' Special Services Program (SSP). The MCCP also serves as a "gate keeper" in prioritizing clients for placement in the various crisis residential beds either publicly or privately administered. It also provides a statewide electronic data base for residential openings.

In the next sections of this chapter, we will provide greater detail about Eastern Minnesota Community Support Services and Mount Olivet Rolling Acres' Special Services Program.

Eastern Minnesota Community Support Services: State-Operated Services

Eastern Minnesota Community Support Services are the state-operated crisis-respite services designed to assist clients whose behavior places them at risk of losing their community residences or vocational placements. The overarching intent is to provide an immediate and cost-effective "safety net" range of behavioral support services for people with developmental disabilities or related conditions. This is achieved by providing a package of specialized behavioral support services combining short-term behavioral consultation, on-site evaluations, direct service provisions, and residential crisis-respite stays.

Minnesota assures that the provision of crisis-respite services will be cost-effective compared with the acute care costs that would have been paid in the absence of the crisis services. The allocation of funding for crisis-respite services is made to regions of the state in an annual plan approved by the Commissioner of Human Services. Crisis services demonstrate ongoing cost-effectiveness by operating within the costs of approved crisis-respite plans and by reducing the use of other acute crisis care.

The overall intervention strategy of EMCSS focuses on eliminating gaps between the client's behavioral competencies and his or her individualized systems of supports. These clinical goals are accomplished by designing and delivering an individualized package of clinical crisis services for the recipient that may include:

1. Assessment to determine the precipitating factors contributing to the crisis situation.

2. Development of a coordinated intervention plan.

3. Behavioral consultation and staff training to the care providers to ensure successful implementation.

4. Development and implementation of a transition plan to assist the client in returning home if temporary residential treatment was provided.

5. Ongoing technical assistance to the care providers in the implementation of the intervention plan developed for the client.

6. Development of a crisis support plan to prevent or minimize future crisis situations and increase the likelihood of maintaining the client in his or her community.

Eligibility Criteria

The following criteria must be met for a client to receive crisis-respite services:

1. The care providers have been unable to provide the necessary interventions and protection of the client or others.

2. The provision of the crisis-respite services will enable the client to avoid acute crisis care placement.

3. The temporary residential treatment should not exceed 90 days.

4. The client has been screened and authorized as eligible to receive home and community-based waivered services.

Unlike other waivered services, the crisis-respite service must be immediately available to the client as an alternative to acute crisis care placements.

Whether public- or private-sector, all providers of crisis services seeking Medicaid waiver funding must have a current provider agreement with their local county agencies. The provider agreement specifies the county agencies' responsibilities, crisis-respite service providers' responsibilities, the services to be provided, the network of specialized service providers to be used, the projected annual costs, how utilization and effectiveness will be monitored and reported, and how the Medicaid cost-effectiveness of the crisis-respite services will be assured.

Special Services Program: Private-Operated Services

In 1992, the Minnesota state legislature responded to a request from various county and community agencies by authorizing funding for a private community-based crisis intervention service. This program, called the Special Services Program, was located within an existing intermediate care facility (Mount Olivet Rolling Acres) for people with mental retardation in a suburb of Minneapolis. It was to serve five counties in the western Minneapolis metropolitan area. The legislature established two goals for this program. The first was to prevent acute crisis care placements due to behavioral crises and, when necessary, provide a temporary residential treatment alternative to costly psychiatric hospitalizations or regional center placements. The second goal was to keep clients in their homes and communities at equal or lower costs than would have been expended for institutional care.

Like public crisis services, the SSP provides two types of crisis prevention and response services. The first is community outreach to clients concerning behavior, health, and psychiatric diagnosis and treatment. The second type of crisis service provided is a short-term (i.e., up to 90 days) residential stay in a four-bed unit with enriched staffing (1-to-2 staff-client ratio). Both services involve multidisciplinary planning and intervention focused on a functional assessment and a nonaversive response to challenging behavior. Whenever possible, outreach interventions and supports are promoted as the first choice of services. Generally, they are offered to individuals with the greatest risk of losing their community placements.

The goal for the comprehensive assessment is a thorough understanding of the client's abilities, his or her medical conditions and treatments, mental health needs, communicative abilities, and the functions of the challenging behaviors. Also included are a description of their past and current residential and day placements coupled with an analysis of the social and physical environment that may be contributing to the challenging behaviors. This assessment is conducted through (a) direct observation of the client at home and work or school; (b) individual and group interviews with county case manager, family members, and service providers; and (c) a careful review of the client's written records (e.g., vocational services or educational plans, psychological, psychiatric, and other medical reports). The crisis team assimilates both verbal and written information relevant to each client's behavior and the various contributing factors. Areas assessed include social interaction and communication; environmental, medical, and psychiatric factors; personal preferences and reinforcement histories; and a functional assessment of target behaviors.

The product of this assessment is a detailed report that provides demographic and referral information, a description of the data collected and the sources of information, a review of the client's strengths and abilities, the individual's residential history, vocational placement, physical and mental health review, definitions of the challenging behaviors, the hypothesized motivational functions of the challenging behaviors, an environmental analysis, and the intervention recommendations. The treatment recommendations are divided into areas concerning direct treatment or intervention (e.g., medication adjustments or other behavioral strategies that may have more immediate impact on the behavior); positive programming (i.e., longer-term skills training or therapy strategies); environmental modifications (i.e., physical and social changes); and reactive or emergency strategies, staff and care provider training, data collection, and follow-up.

Care provider training entails verbal and written instructions as well as modeling and role-playing exercises. The special-services staff, either directly, indirectly, or through other community specialists, provide educational materials and training on issues relevant to clients' families and service providers (e.g., communication strategies, sensory integration, techniques and treatments for particular psychiatric diagnoses). Ongoing consultation is provided regarding specific environmental modifications, behavioral interventions, or the implementation of other treatment approaches.

Similarities Between Public and Private Crisis Services

As is evident, close similarities exist between the public and private providers' crisis services. Both services share the same goals and provide both outreach technical assistance and short-term 24-hour crisis-respite care.

Both EMCSS and SSP evolved from previous intermediate care facilities for people with mental retardation (ICF-MR). The services of EMCSS emanate from the Minnesota Extended Treatment Options (further described below), and MCCP and SSP are administered through Mount Olivet Rolling Acres. Because prevention of more restrictive placements is a fundamental goal, both employ nonaversive behavioral support strategies to ensure ongoing successful living in the community.

The collaborative nature of the public and private crisis service providers prevent a competitive relationship. On a practical day-to-day level, staff members from both crisis-service public and private sectors may conjointly provide services to the client. For example, one behavior analyst may conduct a functional assessment, while the treatment strategies are developed through consultation with employees of both sectors.

The following is a case example that describes the outreach component of crisis services with a possible placement in a temporary residential treatment facility.

Case Example[2]

This is an example of a fictitious person, Linda, who is in her midtwenties. This client is representative of the technical assistance outreach component provided by both the state and private sector employees.

The county case manager contacted the Metro Crisis Coordination Program, inquiring about assistance. The client, Linda, refused to attend her supported employment site and appeared to be having tantrums at the workshop where she arrived each morning. After the intake information was obtained, decisions were necessary. Should either the private or public outreach component serve as the primary clinical service provider? Should both work together for a more rapid response? Or would the case be better served by a practitioner outside the domain of crisis prevention and response? It was determined that a state behavior analyst

---

[2] This case example is representative of a number of clients served in the Minneapolis-St. Paul area. A fictitious client is used to ensure that real clients are neither identified nor identifiable.

would provide initial consultation services. MCCP asked whether the facility needed augmentative staffing, from either the public or private sector, to work with the technical assistance consultant in providing direct care for 2 weeks to assist the client in the de-escalation of crisis behavior.

Initially, the behavior analyst interviewed the foster parents, the program director of the worksite, and the job coach. In consultation with the county case manager, it was determined that augmentative staffing was not necessary. What was needed was an intervention strategy for day program staff to follow in decreasing Linda's tantrums and gain her cooperation to work off-site.

The first step was for the behavior analyst to conduct functional assessment interviews with the foster parents, case manager, program director, and job coach at Linda's worksite. This interview employed the questionnaire developed by O'Neill et al. (1997). The foster parents reported on Linda's behavior prior to leaving for her day program and upon returning from work. The case manager reviewed Linda's general living history, parental and family involvement, and the results of previous programmatic interventions. The staff at the worksite described Linda's behavior at work and what strategies they implemented to ameliorate her problem behaviors.

The results of this assessment were used to identify the setting events that altered the evoking properties of antecedent events and the reinforcing quality of the consequences. Identification of the antecedents and consequences of the problem behavior was also important. Each member of Linda's interdisciplinary team provided valuable information for the completion of this functional assessment.

The results suggested multiple causation of Linda's problem behavior. She was able to avoid going to her job site (a negative reinforcement component), she was able to receive encouragement from foster parents and staff to work at her job site (a positive reinforcement component), and she was able to participate in daily alternative tasks at the home work station.

The foster parents reported they had a positive relationship with Linda and that other than some idiosyncratic events, which are upsetting to her, she was pleasant, cooperative, and appeared to enjoy participating in activities at home. The case manager described Linda's work history and the difficulties Linda had experienced that resulted in repeated dismissals from previous worksites. Past reactive strategies included timeout, enforced relaxation, and manual restraint contingent on the emission of her tantrums, subsequent to her refusal to work. The staff from her employment site reported Linda enjoyed the enriched individual attention she received from working and the staff-client ratio, which was generally one staff for two clients. For this reason, they were perplexed why Linda continued having tantrums and refusing to work off-site.

The behavior analyst decided to observe Linda when she arrived at her worksite. It was the worksite's policy that each client, regardless of level of functioning, would not be required to participate in his or her work program. It was considered the client's individual decision even though work staff may encourage participation, they did not require it.

When the behavior analyst observed Linda and the staff response to her work refusal, a number of salient environmental events became evident. When Linda had a tantrum, staff were always nearby to provide comfort. After her tantrum subsided and the supported employment staff left the work station, Linda visited other staff members who freely interacted with her. These staff were generally cheerful men who joked and teased with her. One staff person reported that Linda was really a fun person after her daily tantrums subsided.

It became evident that staff, albeit well-intentioned, were inadvertently reinforcing her work refusal and tantrum episodes. A behavior support plan reversing this situation proved successful in decreasing these problem behaviors. That is, the essential component of the plan was to provide enhanced recognition for work at her scheduled supported employment site and planned ignoring of her work refusal.

Although positive results occurred in this case, the question arises about what if all the outreach services had been ineffective and Linda's tantrums were not lessened? Moreover, what if her foster parents decided that they would no longer allow Linda to live with them even though she had done so for many years?

In these situations, MCCP could again be contacted to report the unsuccessful outcome. Neither psychiatric hospitalization nor admission to a large congregate facility would be viewed as a desirable option. As a more desirable alternative, MCCP would refer Linda to temporary residential treatment operated either by EMCSS or SSP. This short-term residential placement would provide stabilization and an opportunity to observe her behaviors 24 hours a day and closely evaluate possible treatment strategies. Once Linda returns to her foster home and community worksite, technical assistance would resume to maximize her successful community living.

Linda's problem behaviors did not pose a public safety risk. However, there are clients whose behaviors are so challenging that community crisis services are insufficient and more intensive residential treatment is necessary. In these situations, the final safety net is the Minnesota Extended Treatment Options (METO) program.

METO: Safety-Net Services

METO is a state-operated ICF-MR residential program providing services for adults with intellectual disabilities who are considered a risk to public safety, are in need of active treatment, and do not have an alternative community residential placement able to provide services. The clients admitted to METO are court committed usually due to severe aggressive or destructive behaviors or sexual predation. Located on the grounds of a former regional treatment center (Cambridge Regional Human Services Center), three newly constructed self-contained side-by-side duplexes are in use and one additional building is being constructed for a total of 48 clients. Each of the eight units is designed to be self-contained, having a maximum of six clients per unit with their own private bedrooms. The services are limited to those individuals whose behavior disorders require short-term intervention until their problem behaviors can be safely managed in a community-based program.

Case Example of Client Admitted to METO[3]

This scenario represents composite examples of clients referred to METO. It describes John, a fictitious man in his late twenties. The case manager referred John to the private crisis services for assistance in reducing his aggressive and destructive behavior. This client had a history of severe aggression and, at the time of referral, had severely injured his job coach, causing dismissal from his day treatment and habilitation program. Shortly after crisis services were initiated, John violently attacked his primary care provider at his residence. The residential program director informed the county case manager that the program could no longer continue to serve this client. John's violent behavior continued to escalate, and he was deemed a risk to public safety. The interdisciplinary team decided to hospitalize John in a psychiatric unit and also consider him for admission to the METO program.

John was evaluated by the EMCSS psychologist while in a locked hospital psychiatric unit. At the time he was seen, John was in a seclusion room because he had accosted a nurse who attempted to provide his oral psychotropic medications. His aggressive behavior required hospital security staff to control John by escorting him to the seclusion room.

For the interview, the EMCSS psychologist was accompanied by two male psychiatric technicians who provided additional supervision. Although John was generally calm, he occasionally became expressively angry. While clinching his fist, he belligerently reported he was going to kill his case manager, guardian, and primary caregiver. John lacked insight and did not express any remorse about the past assaults.

Both the case manager and legal guardian reported that John had previously threatened to injure them. As evident from the assaults to his job coach and his primary care provider, John's verbal threats were credible and considered very serious.

John was court-committed into the METO program, where he received treatment including a behavior support program based on a functional assessment,

---

[3] This fictitious case example represents the collective behavior of a number of different clients. It is presented in this fashion to safeguard the identifiability of individual clients.

medication adjustments, anger management training, and both individual and group psychotherapy. Once John is no longer considered a public safety risk and a community-based residential placement secured, he will be discharged. At the point of his return to community living, both the public and private support services will continue assisting John in his transition to community living.

Some Potential Barriers to a Public-Private Collaboration

A number of issues in the collaboration between the public and private sectors need consideration. Historically, the *state sector* referred to staff working in Minnesota state regional treatment centers. The *private sector* referred to staff working in community-based smaller facilities for people with intellectual disabilities. Throughout the deinstitutionalization movement, state regional centers took on a pejorative connotation that often generalized to the staff offering care for their clients. On the other hand, community-based facilities were viewed as positive, and this connotation generalized to the staff working at these sites. Overcoming this history of working independently of each other represented a major challenge for the development of a collaboration between the state and private sectors. With continued efforts among agencies, many of the barriers have been addressed, as evident in the similarities of the service options previously described.

The wage discrepancy between the public- and private-sector employees could also be a potential barrier. The public sector working in state facilities was unionized and paid a higher wage than those in the private sector. Historically, the private sector received a wage approximately two thirds that of the staff in the public sector (*Association of Residential Resources v. Gomez,* 1994).

The collaborative interaction between public- and private-sector employees in providing crisis prevention and response services in the Twin City metropolitan area of Minnesota have comparable funding and philosophical substrates of clinical treatment. Services provided are constrained neither by managed care nor the usual procedure codes that Medicaid or Medicare would reimburse. If constraints in funding were different for either the public or private services, a potential barrier might exist. The provider who had to exist with limitations on the services they could provide would likely hinder the collaborative relationship between the two sectors.

Philosophical differences in how to provide services could severely hamper the public-private collaboration. This difference is most notable when comparing traditional interventions with those based on the features of positive behavioral support. Carr (1999) describes five fundamental points of contrast that are apparent between the two approaches.

First, the traditional approach focuses on crisis management; the positive behavior support approach stresses prevention. As a result, the traditional approach primarily concerns reactive strategies, whereas the positive behavioral approach emphasizes a comprehensive functional assessment and a support plan to prevent the occurrence of behavioral crises.

Second, the traditional approach examines the topographical features of the problem behavior; the positive behavioral support approach focuses on the hypothesized motivational functions of the target behaviors. The traditional approach addresses each behavior disturbance with separate interventions. For example, there might be one specific reactive strategy for physical aggression and another for verbal threatening. The positive behavioral support approach identifies response classes of the problem behaviors, that is, topographically dissimilar behaviors with similar functional properties.

Third, the traditional approach seeks to suppress the problem behavior; the positive behavioral support approach emphasizes education and skill building. Very frequently, the traditional approach of suppressing the problem behaviors results in using aversive consequences without developing socially appropriate replacement behaviors. The educational and skill-building features of positive behavioral support require a thorough functional assessment to identify the motivational properties of problem behaviors. The educational component emphasizes teaching the client a functionally equivalent response that makes the problem behavior irrelevant, inefficient, and ineffective (Horner, Albin, Sprague, & Todd, 1999).

Fourth, the traditional approach is generally individual-client oriented; the positive behavioral approach tends to be system oriented. That is, the traditional approach focuses on problem behaviors as evidence of an individual's underlying disorder and results in strategies to discourage the client from displaying these behaviors. The positive behavioral support approach generally considers problem behaviors as the result of the environmental context. With this approach, the goal is to alter the systems in which the individual lives to enrich the person's lifestyle quality, thereby obviating the need to display problem behaviors.

Finally, the traditional approach is viewed as molecular in nature; the positive behavioral support being molar (Carr, Carlson, Langdon, Magito-McLaughlin, & Yarbrough, 1998). The traditional approach identifies specific problem behaviors and addresses behavior management programs to suppress these particular behaviors. The positive behavioral support approach is molar; it attends to widespread and diverse lifestyle changes. Fundamentally, this functional approach searches for methods to remediate deficient physical and social environments, thus making the display of problem behaviors less likely.

Fortunately, the public-private sectors providing crisis services in the Twin City metro area of Minnesota both adhere to the positive behavioral support approach. However, if a lack of agreement existed in philosophies of care and treatment, this would severely hamper the public-private collaboration.

Greater Minnesota: The Emerging Development of Public and Private Crisis Services

The initial proposal of outreach crisis services occurred in 1988. In 1992 legislation authorizing crisis services through pilot projects was approved. By 1993 statewide crisis services were either being provided or in the process of development. The public-private collaboration has also occurred in other regions of Minnesota. For example, Providers of South-East Minnesota (ProSEM) is a private agency working in conjunction with EMCSS. The model is similar to what was developed in the Twin City metro region.

The Minnesota outcome research in facilitating deinstitutionalization and preventing institutionalization in the metro area of Minnesota has been presented elsewhere (Colond & Wieseler, 1995; Hanson, Oslund, & Wieseler, 1997; Rudolph et al., 1998). The nationwide accelerating trend of deinstitutionalization beckons for crisis services development in other locations. The success Minnesota has experienced in its public and private collaboration is worthy for consideration when developing similar services in other state.

References

Anderson, L. L., Lakin, K. C., Mangan, T. W., & Prouty, R. W. (1998). State institutions: Thirty years of depopulation and closure. *Mental Retardation, 36,* 431–443.

Association of Residential Resources v. Gomez, 94–1801, 94–1865, 94–2432 (District of MN, 1994).

Beasley, J., Kroll, J., & Sovner, R. (1992). Community-based crisis mental health services for persons with developmental disabilities: The S.T.A.R.T. model. *Habilitative Mental Healthcare Newsletter, 11,* 55–57.

Carr, E. G. (1999, May). *Positive behavioral supports: Philosophy, methods, and outcomes.* Paper presented at the Scott Doss Memorial Conference on Positive Behavioral Supports in the Community, Home, and School, Minneapolis, MN.

Carr, E. G., Carlson, J. I., Langdon, N. A., Magito-McLaughlin, D., & Yarbrough, S. C. (1998). Two perspectives on antecedent control: Molecular and Molar. In J. K. Luiselli & M. J. Cameron (Eds.), *Antecedent control: Innovative approaches to behavioral support* (pp. 3–28). Baltimore: Paul H. Brookes.

Carr, E. G., Levin, L., McConnachie, G., Carlson, J. I., Kemp, D. C., Smith, C. E., & McLaughlin, D. M. (1999). Comprehensive multisituational intervention for problem behavior in the community: Long-term maintenance and social validation. *Journal of Positive Behavior Interventions, 1,* 5–25.

Colond, J. S., & Wieseler, N. A. (1995). Preventing restrictive placements through Community Support Services. *American Journal on Mental Retardation, 100,* 201–206.

Davidson, P. W., Cain, N. N., Sloan-Reeves, J. E., Giesow, V. E., Quijano, L. E., Van Heyningen, J., & Shoham, H. (1995). Crisis intervention for community-based individuals with developmental disabilities and behaviors and psychiatric disorders. *Mental Retardation, 33,* 21–2–30.

Fitzpatrick, T. (1995). *National trends in serving individuals with severe behaviors.* Minneapolis: University of Minnesota Institute on Community Integration, unpublished manuscript.

Hanson, R. H., Oslund, J. M., & Wieseler, N. A. (1997). Crisis services for persons with dual diagnosis in Minnesota. *NADD (National Association for the Dually Diagnosed) Newsletter, 14,* 69–70.

Horner, R. H., Albin, R. W., Sprague, J. R., & Todd, A. W. (1999). Positive behavior support. In M. E. Snell & F. Brown (Eds.), *Instruction of Students With Severe Disabilities* (5th ed.) (pp. 207–244). Upper Saddle River, NJ: Prentice Hall.

Intagliata, J., & Willer, B. (1982). Deinstitutionalization of mentally retarded persons successfully placed into family-care and group homes. *American Journal of Mental Deficiency, 87,* 34–39.

Jacobson, J. W., & Schwartz, A. A. (1983). Personal and service characteristics affecting group home placement success: A prospective analysis. *Mental Retardation, 22,* 231–239.

Lakin, K. C., Hayden, M. F., & Abery, B. H. (1994). An overview of the community living concept. In M. F. Hayden & B. H. Abery (Eds.), *Challenges for a service system in transition: Ensuring quality community experiences for persons with developmental disabilities* (pp. 3–22). Baltimore: Paul H. Brookes.

Nord, G., Wieseler, N. A., & Hanson, R. H. (1997). The assessed crisis services needs of clients in community-based programs serving persons with developmental disabilities. *Behavioral Interventions, 13,* 169–179.

O'Neill, R. E., Horner, R. H., Albin, R. W., Sprague, J. R., Storey, K., & Newton, J. S. (1997). *Functional assessment and program development for problem behavior: A practical handbook.* New York: Brooks/Cole.

Pfadt, A., & Holburn, C. S. (1996). Community-based support services update. *Habilitative Mental Healthcare Newsletter, 15,* 8–11.

Rudolph, C. E., Lakin, K. C., Oslund, J. M., & Larson, W. (1998). Evaluation of outcomes and cost-effectiveness of a community behavioral support and crisis response demonstration project. *Mental Retardation, 36,* 187–197.

Scheerenberger, R. C. (1981). Deinstitutionalization: Trends and difficulties. In R. H. Bruininks, C. E. Meyers, B. B. Sigford, & K. C. Lakin (Eds.), *Deinstitutionalization and community adjustment of mentally retarded people* (pp. 3–13). Washington, DC: American Association on Mental Deficiency.

Schroeder, S. R., Rojahn, J., & Oldenquist, A. (1989). *Treatment of destructive behaviors among people with developmental disabilities: Overview of the problem.* Background paper prepared for the National Institute of Health Consensus Development Panel and the Treatment of Destructive Behavior. Bethesda, MD: National Institute of Health.

Sovner, R., & DesNoyers Hurley, A. (1988). The community residence psychiatric interface. *Psychiatric Aspects of Mental Retardation Reviews, 7,* 52–59.

CHAPTER 5

Behavioral and Crisis Services in California

Gregory A. Wagner
California Department of Developmental Services
Sacramento, California

In both institutional and community settings, challenging behavior presents numerous problems for people with developmental disabilities and for people who provide services and supports. These problems range from behavior that is primarily a nuisance to others, interferes with learning, or results in stigmatization, to behavior that causes injury or death. Challenging behavior, particularly aggression and property destruction, is also a frequent cause of more-restrictive placements (Davidson et al., 1995; Eyman & Call, 1977; Keys, Boroskin, & Ross, 1973; Lakin, Hill, Hauber, Bruininks, & Heal, 1983; Landesman-Dwyer & Sulzbacher, 1981; Mayeda & Sutter, 1981; Pagel & Whitling, 1978; Scheerenberger, 1981; Sutter, Mayeda, Call, Yanagi, & Yee, 1980).

Institutional settings are typically somewhat insular relative to the communities within which they are located. These settings are often able to tolerate a greater severity and magnitude of challenging behavior by virtue of this insularity (Lowe & Felce, 1995). Relatedly, researchers have found higher use of crisis intervention in community settings relative to institutional settings (Stancliffe, Hayden, & Lakin, 1999). With increasing rates of deinstitutionalization, resulting institutional closures, and mandates to use nonrestrictive, "socially valid" procedures to manage and treat challenging behavior, community settings have come under increasing pressures to support people with challenging behavior in the least restrictive means possible. Kormann (1997) captured this reality by noting, "The end of the 20th century brings with it a variety of societal and sociopolitical changes within the field of developmental disabilities. None seems more complex than the movement toward full community participation of individuals with significant psychiatric and behavioral needs" (p. 4).

These realities are no different in California than anywhere else in the country. Indeed, recent events have exacerbated these issues in California. These events include a class action lawsuit that increased the rate of deinstitutionalization and resulted in institutional closures. The current chapter describes the California service system and current demographics of the population served; the recent deinstitutionalization activities and consequences with regard to community behavioral and crisis supports, including criminal justice issues; and concludes with descriptions of some model programs and a discussion of the role of behavior analysis in the provision of effective services.

Organization of the California Service System

The California service system for people with developmental disabilities is governed by the Lanterman Developmental Disabilities Services Act, the original version of which was written in 1969. This law entitles all people with developmental disabilities in the state to receive appropriate services, and it provided for the creation of a statewide regional center system. Currently the regional center system consists of 21 private, nonprofit locally based centers with which the state contracts. These regional centers are the point of entry into the developmental services system for the 58 counties in California. Their role in the system is to coordinate services and supports through generic agencies or directly fund services and supports. In addition to individualized planning and service coordination, services provided directly by regional centers include assessment and diagnosis, information and referral, advocacy, and resource development. The full range of community living options are provided, operated by regional center vendors. The state directly administers five institutions (developmental centers) and two smaller, specialized behavioral facilities, each serving 55 to 65 people.

In the latter 1980s, regional resource development projects (RRDPs) were created at each developmental center, to assist regional centers in developing and enhancing services and supports for consumers moving into community settings. These RRDPs each consist of several state employees who serve a number of roles with respect to developing and enhancing services and supports. For example, these projects monitor people placed from developmental centers into community settings for the first year of placement; they provide a variety of community training opportunities; and they provide and/or assist in securing and coordinating needed clinical services.

Current Demographics

Currently the system serves more than 170,000 people, fewer than 3,800 of whom are served in the state's congregate facilities. Table 5.1 compares people who reside in community settings and people who reside in the five developmental centers across a number of behavioral and psychiatric characteristics. These data are based on a July 2000 summary of the *Client Developmental Evaluation Report* (California Department of Developmental Services, 1978), completed annually for all consumers in developmental centers and triannually for all consumers in community settings.

The data in Table 5.1 show that people residing in developmental centers have substantially higher rates of challenging behavior and psychiatric diagnoses than people living in community settings. These data are consistent with recent data collected elsewhere (e.g., Sturmey & Adams, 1999). Thus a significant number of people currently living in California developmental centers will present an ongoing challenge with respect to successful community placement.

Deinstitutionalization

The history of deinstitutionalization in California is very similar to national trends with regard to overall rate. Figure 5.1 depicts the long-term history of California developmental center census.

As seen in Figure 5.1, the developmental center census remained relatively constant from 1987 to 1992. In 1990 a class-action lawsuit (*Coffelt v. DDS*) was

TABLE 5.1

Behavioral Characteristics of Consumers Residing in California Developmental Centers and Community Settings

Developmental Center	Characteristics	Community
35.5%	Have severe behavioral problems	6.3%
40.8%	Are frequently violent	11.3%
42.9%	Are self-injurious	12.6%
39.0%	Often destroy property	10.3%
54.3%	Have unacceptable social behavior	21.4%
34.1%	Will run away	14.6%
37.0%	Are dually diagnosed	8.4%

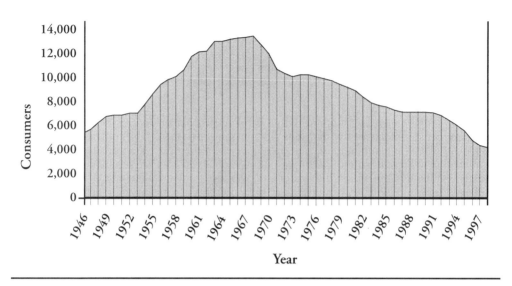

Figure 5.1. California developmental centers census by years.

filed against the California Department of Developmental Services and four regional centers, alleging that too few community living arrangements were being created, resulting in people residing in unnecessarily restrictive institutional settings. This lawsuit was settled in 1994. A major requirement of the resulting settlement was the reduction in developmental center population by 2,000 people (from approx. 6,000) in a 5-year period (1993–1998). This reduction actually took place in 2.5 years, well ahead of schedule. In the process, two developmental centers were closed.

Crisis and Behavioral Support Services

The increased rate of placement resulting from the *Coffelt* (1994) settlement put increased pressures on community crisis and behavioral support systems. In anticipation of these pressures, the settlement included provisions for enhanced crisis intervention services. These provisions required each of the 21 regional centers to develop crisis service proposals. The proposals were based on an initial assessment of local and regional, public or private emergency and crisis services, and corresponding gaps in each geographic area. In addition, crisis proposals were developed through collaborative meetings with relevant agencies (e.g., mental health), providers, and consumers. Finally, the respective roles and responsibilities of the various agencies involved in providing crisis intervention services were delineated (i.e., who is responsible for providing and/or paying for specific services). Plans included provisions for crisis intervention teams, emergency housing, and regional center after-hours response systems. The primary emphasis of these services was "to maintain persons . . . in the living arrangements of their own choice. If dislocation cannot be avoided, every effort will be made to return the person to his or her living arrangement of choice, with all necessary supports, as soon as possible" (*Coffelt v. DDS*, 1993, III, E,1.).

In 1998 many of these and other provisions were written into law. For example, if a consumer's placement is failing and admission to a developmental center is likely, the state must arrange for an immediate assessment of the situation and ensure that the responsible regional center provides necessary emergency services and supports, and convenes an individual program plan as soon as possible. Additional language was written into law, with a focus on people with dual diagnosis. These requirements included memoranda of understanding (MOUs) between each of the 21 regional centers and the local county mental health agencies. These MOUs: (a) identify staff in both agencies who are responsible for identifying consumers with dual diagnosis "of mutual concern," and coordinating services for those people; (b) include a crisis intervention plan with after-hours emergency response capability; (c) include procedures for joint clinical and discharge planning for people admitted to inpatient mental health facilities; and (d) provide for training of residential and day program staff regarding effective services for people with dual diagnosis. In addition, these MOUs are to be reviewed for effectiveness in meeting local needs, by the respective agencies, at least annually. A report describing these MOUs, availability of mobile crisis intervention services, and emergency housing options is provided to the legislature each year.

Within these general systemic requirements of emergency and crisis services outlined above, a variety of specific preventive and reactive strategies have been implemented. Indeed, the sheer size and geographic diversity of California requires varying arrays of services and supports based on differing needs and resources. Following are some examples of specific strategies and activities:

- Some regional centers have developed consumer "risk profiles" to assist case managers and providers in predicting and intervening at early stages of potential behavioral crises. These profiles include environmental antecedents and behavioral precursors predictive of crises.

- Regional centers often maintain lists of behaviorally high-risk consumers, with pertinent information on effective strategies with each consumer and local crisis and emergency services. This information is typically provided to on-call staff via laptop computers.

- Regional centers commonly hold routine multidisciplinary staff meetings to identify at-risk consumers, develop individual crisis plans for those consumers, and problem-solve current difficult cases (e.g., consumers who are at risk of relocation, especially admission to a developmental center; incarcerated; in a psychiatric hospital; etc). In addition, some centers have internal "intensive support services units" or "precrisis screening teams" devoted to these issues.

• Many regional centers provide enhanced case management (i.e., reduced case loads) for consumers who have been recently placed into community settings from developmental centers or have extremely challenging behavior.

• While regional centers primarily coordinate and/or broker necessary services and supports, recent increased funding has provided for the addition of clinical teams to the centers, allowing for the provision of increased direct services by regional centers staff (e.g., behavioral, medical, psychiatric). Also regional center vendors (i.e., behavior analysts, pharmacists, psychiatrists, etc., including university-affiliated programs) provide additional clinical services.

• In addition to regional center staff and vendors, state development center and regional resource project staff provide clinical outreach services (e.g., behavioral consultation, medication review), training (e.g., managing aggressive behavior, teaching new skills) and technical assistance (e.g., meeting regulatory requirements, obtaining needed resources). Also, developmental centers have developed university-based psychology internship programs, wherein psychology interns, under the guidance and supervision of a developmental center psychologist, provide assistance both in transitioning people into the community, and in community behavioral services for consumers whose challenging behavior threatens their placement. These services include functional assessments, development of behavioral plans and strategies, direct therapeutic interactions, and staff training and consultation.

• Interagency collaborative meetings are held in some parts of the state, with participants from regional centers, mental health, criminal justice, and so forth. Training opportunities, workshops, and seminars are provided to those agencies, as well as to providers and families regarding behavioral, psychiatric, and crisis issues.

• Telemedicine (e.g., psychiatric and psychotropic medication consultations) has been effectively incorporated into some rural locations, and its use continues to increase.

• Enhanced staffing (including one-to-ones with corresponding plans to fade the staff) may be used.

• Peer mentors have been arranged for providers and families with behaviorally challenging consumers.

• Person-centered planning is now required by law as a framework for developing IPPs.

To evaluate the overall quality of services and supports and consumer satisfaction with those services and supports during the implementation of the Coffelt (1994) settlement, a longitudinal study of a sample of class members was conducted. (Recent amendments to the Lanterman Developmental Disabilities Services Act require that a similar study continue indefinitely.) Part of this evaluation included annual analyses of mental health and crisis service utilization. Table 5.2 summarizes use of mental health services (e.g., counseling), psychotropic medication consultation, and crisis services across several years of the settlement period. These data show that the use of mental health services varied from 26% to 48% per year and decreased each year from 1996 to 1998. Similarly, psychotropic medication consults ranged from 12% to 26% per year and decreased each year. Finally, between 8% and 17% of the samples received crisis services. Reasons for the wide ranges and decreases over time with respect to mental health and psychotropic medication services are not clear.

Not surprisingly, the people receiving the above services tended to be relatively higher functioning with substantially more challenging behavior than the other class members. A small group of consumers — 3.1% in Conroy, Seiders, Yuskauskas, and Elks (1997) and 4% in Seiders and Conroy (1998) — spent at least one night away from their home due to crises. A small percentage of people also

TABLE 5.2

Mental Health and Crisis Services Use for Samples of People Who Moved From California Institutions to Community Settings

Study	N	Received mental health services	Psychotropic medication review and/or adjustment	Received crisis services
Conroy, 1996	438	47%	26%	—
Conroy, Seiders, Yuskauskas, & Elks, 1997	774	35%	22%	12%
Seiders & Conroy, 1998	1,159	26%	12%	8%
Strong, Almandsmith, Freeman, & Shea, 1998	891	48%	—	17%

indicated needs for greater access to mental health counseling or therapy, including access to psychiatrists, and adjustment of psychotropic medications. Finally, with respect to reported satisfaction with behavioral and crisis services, "supplemental supports" (e.g., in-home behavioral consultation and intervention, enhanced staffing, etc.) and regional center after-hours phone response tended to get the highest ratings across years, while incarceration and emergency rooms received the lowest ratings.

Criminal Justice Issues and Activities

In addition to community crisis and behavioral support activities, criminal justice issues in California are receiving increased attention with respect to identifying and providing appropriate services and supports. As for current activities regarding this population, the California Department of Corrections, with 33 prisons and nearly 140,000 prisoners, has recently settled a lawsuit (*Clark v. State of California,* 1997) alleging that at least 2,500 people with developmental disabilities within the prison system were not receiving adequate accommodations, protection, and services. The Department of Corrections agreed to identify prisoners with developmental disabilities (with an initial screening and, if indicated, a subsequent full evaluation) and to ensure adequate support services for these people, including staff training, access to education, vocational, medical, and other services, and appropriate housing in a secure setting. An anticipated outcome of this settlement is increased awareness, by courts, of the issues, and a resulting increase in the number of people with developmental disabilities identified early in the criminal justice process and diverted to the developmental services system. Increased attention to criminal justice issues has led to the following actions in both community and institutional settings.

Within community settings, recent amendments to the Lanterman Developmental Disabilities Services Act (1969, amended 2001) require each regional center to have "criminal justice expertise to assist the regional center in providing services and support to consumers involved in the criminal justice system as a victim, defendant, inmate or parolee." In addition, efforts have increased throughout the 21 regional centers to identify people with developmental disabilities as soon as they get in trouble with the law, and to work with criminal justice personnel to develop plans and solutions other than jail or prison, such as diversion or probation arrangements.

A major example of criminal justice efforts is a project involving the seven regional centers in the Los Angeles area. Originally created in 1975 and coordinated by South Central Los Angeles Regional Center since 1979, a law enforcement liaison position is stationed in the county jail, to serve all seven Los Angeles County regional centers. This position coordinates services for inmates with developmental disabilities, prevents inappropriate incarceration, and trains deputies, medical staff, and mental health staff in how to identify people with developmental disabilities and how to refer for appropriate regional center services. In 1997 forensic services were expanded under a grant to South Central Los Angeles Regional Center to serve consumers of all seven Los Angeles County regional centers. These services include: (a) a multiagency advisory board to enhance interagency coordination and resource exchange, with members from 20 different agencies (e.g., law enforcement, mental health, Los Angeles County regional centers, courts); (b) training for the various agencies (e.g., education, providers, mental health staff, law enforcement, lawyers, regional center staff) regarding developmental disabilities, the criminal justice system, regional center system, and community services and resources; and (c) a juvenile liaison position to assist in identifying people with developmental disabilities in juvenile hall and to coordinate appropriate services. The juvenile liaison also coordinates preventive interventions for at-risk and predelinquent youths, working with schools, regional centers, probation, and California Youth Authority. Finally, a multidisciplinary forensic assessment team was created, consisting of psychologists, a psychiatrist, adult and juvenile law enforcement liaisons, project staff, and others as needed. This team meets weekly to review cases and develop individual justice plans. Recommendations regarding competency, due process, diversion, mental health, and other treatment and clinical issues are made, and follow-up activities conducted. These activities include consultation with specialized drug and alcohol treatment programs, and therapy programs for sex offenders.

The findings from this project indicate that programs that "provide frequent, consistent counseling regarding appropriate behavior," positive consequences for "responsible, crime free behavior," and negative consequences for "dangerous, uncooperative behavior" work best. Also, specialized treatment for drugs, alcohol, and sex offenses are critical, as is involvement in a structured, daily school or work program (South Central Los Angeles Regional Center, 1998).

Within institutional settings, additional activities have occurred. In response to community concerns regarding violent actions of some consumers, recent law requires that individuals charged with a violent felony may be placed only in a facility with a secured perimeter or in a locked and controlled treatment facility. Locked community facilities for people with developmental disabilities don't exist in California. In addition, many community providers have exhausted their ability to create community options for people with very severe challenging behavior and/or dual diagnosis. Indeed, in studying a 1995 institutional closure in California, researchers found that people with dual diagnosis and people with a combination of aggression and criminal justice involvement had the most trouble with respect to community placement. Multiple placements, including psychiatric hospitals and return to developmental centers, were not uncommon for these two groups (Business Services Group, 1998).

The factors described above have led to increased court commitments of people with very challenging behavior and/or criminal justice involvement to developmental centers; they've raised a related challenge to balance security, least restrictive placement, and appropriate treatment. To ensure proper security within the centers, consumers receive an evaluation assessing the person's risk of elopement and risk of dangerous behavior in the community (e.g., sex crimes, property destruction, aggression, burglary, arson) by looking at history, current stressors, mental illness, and so forth. Then, based on a combination of this score and interdisciplinary review and discussion, the person's placement with regard to level of security is determined. These consumers receive an IPP and related services, which may include competency training, educational and vocational services, social skills training (e.g., communication, assertion, and anger management), substance abuse training, sexuality training, victim awareness, and problem solving (Marlowe, 1999).

Summary and Conclusions

Serving people with extremely challenging behavior is difficult in any setting. These difficulties are often exacerbated in community settings in which social tolerance may be less than in institutional settings, and the concomitant emphasis on "socially valid," community referenced interventions is heightened. In addition, some restrictive procedures may be permissible in institutional, but not community settings. In California, as elsewhere in the country, these issues have received increased attention as the rate of deinstitutionalization and institutional closure has increased. Community systems have been forced to respond with enhanced behavioral support and crisis services.

The supports and services in California, described in this chapter, share many elements with successful models elsewhere. For example, Minnesota developed outreach community support services to prevent admission of people with challenging behavior into large regional treatment centers (Colond & Wieseler, 1995). These services are provided on site by behavior analysts, and consist of behavioral assessment, development of behavior programs, staff and family training, program evaluation, and follow-up consultation. Results indicated substantial reduction in admissions to institutions, related cost savings, and high levels of satisfaction among consumers of services. Community support services staff have been added to all of Minnesota's regional treatment centers. As discussed in this chapter, California provides very similar services through both regional center clinical staff and vendors and through developmental center staff, including behavioral psychology interns and regional resource development projects.

In addition to regional treatment center community support services, Rudolph,

Lakin, Oslund, and Larson (1998) described a special services program for be-havioral support and crisis services in Minnesota. This program consists of multi-disciplinary outreach services provided on site, and short-term (90 or fewer days) placement for up to four people at a time. Both services provide functional or be-havioral assessment, development of interventions, staff and family training, and follow-up consultation and technical assistance. Outreach services may also in-clude temporary direct care staffing augmentation, if necessary. This program was successful with respect to maintaining community placements, cost savings, and consumer satisfaction, and has since been expanded throughout Minnesota. Again, many components of this program — particularly the outreach services — are similar to behavioral and multidisciplinary services provided in California.

Rudolph et al. (1998) found that 82% of the people served by their project had psychiatric diagnoses. People with dual diagnoses may pose particularly diffi-cult challenges to service systems. A model crisis intervention program in New York for people with dual diagnosis was described by Davidson et al. (1995). This program was comprised of an interdisciplinary crisis team, a continuum for inpa-tient treatment (including psychiatric and a state-operated group home), and cri-sis prevention services, such as staff training and "family-centered case manage-ment." The crisis intervention team served many of the same functions now man-dated by recent California legislation: "Participation in inpatient treatment and discharge planning during acute psychiatric admissions"; follow-up consultation after discharge; "identification of at-risk consumers"; and staff training for devel-opmental disabilities and mental health staff (Davidson et al., p. 24). In addition, the program was developed through "a comprehensive formal assessment of con-sumer, family, and provider needs; and a survey of resources to identify gaps in the existing service system" (p. 24), all elements in California's initial community be-havioral and crisis services development. The authors of the New York project em-phasized the critical importance of facilitating interagency (developmental dis-ability and mental health) communication and access — an issue of national im-portance for people with dual diagnosis. Davidson et al. found that "behavioral interventions" (data collection systems, behavior programs, staff training) were the most frequently provided services. Consumers referred for services tended to be younger, have aggression or self-injury, and resided in a community residential setting rather than a family setting (Vardi, 1996). More recently, intensive outpa-tient mental health services have been shown to reduce subsequent hospitalizations and lengths of stay for 28 people with dual diagnosis (Holden & Neff, 2000).

The relative success of community living arrangements for people with devel-opmental disabilities and very challenging behavior is a function of many vari-ables. Clearly, the match between consumer and residential setting is critical (Davidson et al., 1995). This match may be enhanced, with respect to consumer choices, through thoughtful person-centered planning. Researchers (e.g., Intagliata & Willer, 1982) have also discussed how characteristics of the setting (e.g., increased "experience, competencies and tolerance of community care providers, support available to providers") may enhance the match between consumer and residential setting, and thus positively affect placement outcome (p. 34; see also Sutter, 1980). Other variables likely to impact successful placement include the speed with which crisis teams respond, and the teams' knowledge of both proactive strategies and mental health issues (Nord, Wieseler, & Hanson, 1998).

Both the quality and quantity of behavioral services are also very important with regard to effective behavioral support and crisis services and successful community placement. A multicomponent system for enhancing the quality and quantity of behavioral services in Florida has been described at length (Johnston & Shook, 1987, 1993). In California, several activities have also taken place to improve behavioral service quality, in addition to those discussed elsewhere in this chapter. For example, existing regulations require review by a "qualified professional" of any behavioral plans, in licensed community care facilities, that may cause "pain or trauma." These plans must be technically adequate, derive from a functional assessment, and include procedures for monitoring and implementation, among other requirements. More recent legislation requires direct care staff in community care facilities to receive 70 hours of training, including segments on teaching and positive behavioral supports. Finally, a formal certification process for behavior analysts and associate behavior analysts has been implemented at the national level through the Behavior Analyst Certification Board. This rigorous process was originally developed in Florida (where the process has been in place for 15 years). Many behavior analysts in California (and many other states) now participate in this certification.

In conclusion, the approaches derived from applied behavior analysis have provided tools and technologies to dramatically improve functional life skills and reduce challenging behavior, freeing people with developmental disabilities from unnecessarily restrictive placements and procedures. In California, as well as in the states with model programs described above, behavior analysis has provided the conceptual and technological framework to successfully support people in community settings. Behavioral treatment procedures have become increasingly community referenced, including antecedent or ecological manipulations, and teaching functionally equivalent skills to replace challenging behavior (Wagner, in progress). In addition, complementary roles for behavioral and person-centered approaches have been proposed (Wagner, 1999). Further, current refinements in functional analysis and assessment techniques have dramatically improved the effectiveness of behavioral procedures by permitting accurate identification of behavioral functions and using procedures that match those functions.

Despite the increased effectiveness of, and demand for, behavioral technology, some segments of the developmental disabilities field have recently criticized behavioral approaches as being overly controlling and thus unacceptable. These criticisms are largely based on misunderstanding, semantic confusion, and ideological predisposition. Fortunately, the field has not thrown out the baby with the bath water. The need for effective, "socially valid" behavioral technology will only increase. History has repeatedly shown that behavioral science can successfully assist citizens with developmental disabilities to lead fulfilling lives in community settings. As people continue to move into the community, behavioral science and technology will continue to provide the tools to make those moves successful.

Author Note

Sincere appreciation is extended to the following people for editorial or technical assistance: Ron Huff, Bruce Williams, Carolyn Jackson, John Ellis, Paul Carlton, Paul Verke, and Katie Drake.

The opinions expressed herein do not necessarily reflect those of the California Department of Developmental Services.

References

Business Services Group. (1998). *Longitudinal quality of life study: Phase III* (Rep. to the California Department of Developmental Services). Sacramento: California State University, Sacramento, Business Services Group.

California Department of Developmental Services. (1978). *Client Developmental Evaluation Report.* Sacramento: Author.

California Department of Developmental Services (2001). Lanterman Developmental Disabilities Services Act, Sacramento, CA: Author.

Clark v. State of California, No. 96-16952, WL 525518 (9th Cir. Aug. 27, 1997).

Coffelt v. Department of Developmental Services, No. 91-6401, Cal. Super. Ct., Jan. 19, 1994), MPDLR 185.

Colond, J. S., & Wieseler, N. A. (1995). Preventing restrictive placements through community support services. *American Journal on Mental Retardation,* 100, 201–206.

Conroy, J. W. (1996). *Patterns of community placement II: The first 27 months of the Coffelt settlement* (Rep. to the California Department of Developmental Services). Bryn Mawr, PA: Center for Outcome Analysis.

Conroy, J. W., Seiders, J. X., Yuskauskas, A., & Elks, M. (1997). *Mental health and crisis services for Coffelt class members,* 1996–1997 (Rep. to the California Department of Developmental Services). Bryn Mawr, PA: Center for Outcome Analysis.

Davidson, P. W., Cain, N. N., Sloane-Reeves, J. E., Giesow, V. E., Quijano, L. E., Heyningen, J. V., & Shoham, I. (1995). Crisis intervention for community-based individuals with developmental disabilities and behavioral and psychiatric disorders. *Mental Retardation, 33,* 21–30.

Eyman, R. K., & Call, T. (1977). Maladaptive behavior and community placement of mentally retarded persons. *American Journal of Mental Deficiency, 82,* 137–144.

Holden, P., & Neff, J. A. (2000). Intensive outpatient treatment of persons with mental retardation and psychiatric disorder: A preliminary study. *Mental Retardation, 38,* 27–32.

Intagliata, J., & Willer, B. (1982). Reinstitutionalization of mentally retarded persons successfully placed into family-care and group homes. *American Journal of Mental Deficiency, 87,* 34–39.

Johnston, J. M., & Shook, G. L. (1987). Developing behavior analysis at the state level. *Behavior Analyst, 10,* 199–233.

Johnston, J. M., & Shook, G. L. (1993). Model for the statewide delivery of programming services. *Mental Retardation, 31,* 127–139.

Keys, V., Boroskin, A., & Ross, R. (1973, February). The revolving door in an MR hospital: A study of returns from leave. *Mental Retardation, 11,* 55–56.

Kormann, R. J. (1997, March–April). Behavioral support in the community: How will managed care address it? *American Association on Mental Retardation (AAMR) News and Notes, 10,* 4.

Lakin, K. C., Hill, B. K., Hauber, F. A., Bruininks, R. H., & Heal, L. W. (1983). New admissions and readmissions to a national sample of public residential facilities. *American Journal of Mental Deficiency, 88,* 13–20.

Landesman-Dwyer, S., & Sulzbacher, F. M. (1981). Residential placement and adaptation of severely and profoundly retarded individuals. In R. H. Bruininks, C. E. Meyers, B. B. Sigford, & K. C. Lakin (Eds.), *Deinstitutionalization and community adjustment of mentally retarded people* (pp. 182–194). Washington, DC: American Association on Mental Retardation.

Lowe, K., & Felce, D. (1995). How do caregivers assess the severity of challenging behaviour? A total population study. *Journal of Intellectual Disability Research, 39,* 117–127.

Marlowe, R. A. (1999). *Plan for individuals with forensic or severe behavior needs.* Sacramento: California Department of Developmental Services.

Mayeda, T., & Sutter, P. (1981). Deinstitutionalization: Phase II. In R. H. Bruininks, C. E. Meyers, B. B. Sigford, & K. C. Lakin (Eds.), *Deinstitutionalization and community adjustment of mentally retarded people* (pp. 375–381). Washington, DC: American Association on Mental Retardation.

Nord, G. B., Wieseler, N. A., & Hanson, R. H. (1998). The assessed crisis service needs of clients in community-based programs serving persons with developmental disabilities. *Behavioral Interventions, 13,* 169–179.

Pagel, S. E., & Whitling, C. A. (1978). Readmissions to a state hospital for mentally retarded persons: Reasons for community placement failure. *Mental Retardation, 16,* 164–166.

Rudolph, C., Lakin, K. C., Oslund, J. M., & Larson, W. (1998). Evaluation of outcomes and cost-effectiveness of a community behavioral support and crisis response demonstration project. *Mental Retardation, 36,* 187–197.

Scheerenberger, R. C. (1981). Deinstitutionalization: Trends and difficulties. In R. H. Bruininks, C. E. Meyers, B. B. Sigford, & K. C. Lakin (Eds.), *Deinstitutionalization and community adjustment of mentally retarded people* (pp. 3–13). Washington, DC: American Association on Mental Retardation.

Seiders, J. X., & Conroy, J. W. (1998). *Selected findings of the Coffelt quality tracking project* (Rep. to the California Department of Developmental Services). Bryn Mawr, PA: Center for Outcome Analysis.

South Central Los Angeles Regional Center. (1998). *The Forensic Project* (Final Rep.). Los Angeles: Author.

Stancliffe, R. J., Hayden, M. F., & Lakin, K. C. (1999). Interventions for challenging behavior in residential settings. *American Journal of Mental Retardation, 104,* 364–375.

Strong, M. F., Almandsmith, S., Freeman, A. C., & Shea, J. (1998). *Quality of life for persons with developmental disabilities moving from developmental centers into the community* (Rep. to the California Department of Developmental Services). Oakland, CA: Berkeley Planning Associates.

Sturmey, P., & Adams, C. (1999). Level of need and behavioral needs of persons admitted to institutions in Texas, 1994 to 1998. *Mental Retardation, 37,* 497.

Sutter, P. (1980). Environmental variables related to community placement failure in mentally retarded adults. *Mental Retardation, 18,* 189–191.

Sutter, P., Mayeda, T., Call, T., Yanagi, G., & Yee, S. (1980). Comparison of successful and unsuccessful community-placed mentally retarded persons. *American Journal of Mental Deficiency, 85,* 262–267.

Vardi, I. S., Davidson, P. W., Cain, N. N., Sloane-Reeves, J. E., Giesow, V. E., Quijano, L. E., & Houser, K. D. (1996). Factors predicting re-referral following crisis intervention for community-based persons with developmental disabilities and behavioral and psychiatric disorders. *American Journal on Mental Retardation, 101,*109–117.

Wagner, G. A. (1999). Further comments on person-centered approaches. *Behavior Analyst, 22,* 53–54.

Wagner, G. A. *The enduring contributions of behavioral science.* Manuscript in preparation.

Welfare and Institutions Code (or W & I code), Statutes of 1999, Chapter 146, Section 25, 4640.6, (h), (1).

CHAPTER 6

The START/Sovner Center Program in Massachusetts

Joan B. Beasley
Jeri Kroll
Sovner Center/Greater Lynn Mental Health and
Retardation Association
Danvers, Massachusetts

This chapter begins with a brief analysis of some of the issues confronted by individuals with developmental disabilities and community mental health service needs, and their families and service providers, followed by an overview of START (Systemic, Therapeutic, Assessment, Respite, and Treatment) services in northeast Massachusetts. Originally designed primarily as a service linkage approach to coordinated care for individuals with developmental disabilities and behavioral health care needs, the expanded service system facilitates service linkages and provides specialized services as part of the Robert D. Sovner Behavioral Health Resource Center.

In addition to a description of the program and services, the chapter describes the service population and some service outcomes of interest. The chapter concludes with some of the lessons learned after 10 years of operation.

Background

Inadequate community mental health care affects a number of service populations, such as people with long-term mental health care needs. In most cases high rates of psychiatric inpatient hospitalization and lack of continuity in treatment compliance have been identified as key problems to overcome (Mechanic, 1989).

Many believe that this is the direct result of a system that fails to coordinate the multiple services used by many people with mental illness. Most long-term mental health service users require multiple services such as housing, vocational training, day treatment, inpatient services, and outpatient services (Rochefort, 1993). But the community system often lacks the resources needed to provide a coordinated and comprehensive approach to service delivery, thereby fragmenting care and treatment.

In addition to multiple service use, the experience of people with developmental disabilities and behavioral health care needs is further complicated by the use of multiple service systems. Whereas people with mental illness may receive all of their services from "mental health providers," people with developmental disabilities and behavioral health care needs receive their services from either mental health providers or developmental disability providers, depending on the type of service. Many believe that this further fragments a system of care for people with developmental disabilities and behavioral health care needs (Fletcher, 1993).

Menolascino (1983) recommended a "systematic" approach to the management of behavioral health needs of people with developmental disabilities. As part of the systematic approach, key service elements include: the provision of comprehensive diagnostic evaluations (described later); active family involvement and education; early diagnosis and treatment; vocational habilitative services; residential services; and family support with short-term crisis care facilities to provide back-up and support when needed. Menolascino stressed the need for coordinated services and stated:

> Coordination of the many services needed for individuals with dual diagnoses requires awareness of the various services available in a given community and a professional attitude that permits active collaboration. It necessitates sharing of the overall treatment plan with the retarded individual (when appropriate), the family, and with community resources. Close attention to the clarity and continuity of communication is essential. (p. 51)

This chapter defines coordinated service structures and presents the history and outcomes associated with START, a model program to coordinate behavioral health care for individuals with developmental disabilities in northeast Massachusetts that began in 1989. The underlying philosophy of all coordinated care systems such as START is that services will be most effective when everyone involved in care and treatment is allowed to participate actively in diagnostic and treatment planning, including service-use decisions. For this to occur, collaboration between service providers is needed (MARC, 1995; Rambow & Arnold, 1996).

Coordinated care models offer forums to foster communication between professionals and caregivers; to increase access to professionals for information and education; and to allow all caregivers and care recipients the opportunity for input into service and treatment decisions. The hope is that coordination of services through collaboration will increase the abilities of all members of the system and improve treatment outcomes.

Diagnosis and Treatment Issues for People With Developmental Disabilities and Behavioral Health Care Needs

All of the individuals referred to START have mental retardation. By definition, mental retardation is not a diagnosis of a mental disorder, in spite of its classification in the Diagnostic and Statistical Manual (DSM) (Szymanski, 1977). Mental retardation is diagnosed based on age of onset (prior to age 22) and below-average general intellectual functioning, associated with deficits in adaptive functioning. The behaviors associated with the presence of "behavioral problems" and/or "mental" disorders (illness) are not a direct result of having mental retardation, but rather are influenced by environmental factors and/or the presence of a mental disorder (Menolascino, 1989). Unfortunately, there is a tendency for general psychiatric practitioners to attribute symptoms of a mental disorder to mental retardation, a phenomenon known as "diagnostic overshadowing" (Reiss, Levitan, & McNally, 1982). When this occurs, the diagnosis of mental illness is either overlooked or severely compromised.

The unique presentation of many people with mental retardation often requires special clinical skills in the diagnosis and treatment of mental illness as well as other medical conditions (Borthwick, 1988; Bouras, Kon, & Drummond, 1993; Bregman, 1991; Campbell & Malone, 1991; Criscione, Kastner, Walsh, & Nathanson, 1993; Dosen, 1988; Evangelista, 1988; Jacobson, 1990; Menolascino, Gilson, & Levitas, 1986; Sovner, 1986).

Four Effects of Mental Retardation That Affect Diagnosis of Mental Illness

There are four major effects of mental retardation that influence the diagnosis of a mental illness: intellectual distortion, psychosocial masking, cognitive disintegration, and baseline exaggeration (Sovner, 1986).

Intellectual Distortion

Sovner (1986) refers to intellectual distortion as the inability of an individual with developmental disabilities to think abstractly and communicate verbally. Intellectual distortion undermines the results of a diagnostic interview because a person with developmental disabilities may be unable to respond to questions accurately. General mental health diagnostic instruments rely heavily on the individual's ability to self-report if the practitioner is to elicit specific diagnostic criteria. The inability to articulate internal abstract experiences, as well as the experience of concrete thinking, aphasia, limited vocabulary, and hearing deficits — all these greatly hamper the clinician's ability to use these tools effectively in diagnosing a specific disorder, especially because so much is weighted on the clinical interview (Carlson, 1981; McCracken & Diamond, 1988).

Psychosocial Masking

Sovner (1986) uses the term *psychosocial masking* to describe the effects of developmental disabilities on the content of psychiatric symptoms. The limited knowledge of the world along with the limited life experience of an individual with mental retardation or other developmental disabilities may restrict the detail, range, and richness of delusions and hallucinations they experience. This makes it difficult to determine whether or not someone with developmental disabilities is experiencing a "fear" or a "delusion" (Carlson, 1981).

Cognitive Disintegration

Sovner (1986) uses this term, *cognitive disintegration,* to describe the tendency for some individuals with developmental disabilities to become confused when experiencing serious emotional stress. Unrelated to a mental disorder, individuals with developmental disabilities are predisposed, by organic deficits and concrete coping skills, to become confused when under severe stress. At times, they may regress in their behavioral presentation because they cannot express their needs (Ghazi-uddin, 1988; Matson, 1983; Menolascino, 1983; Revill, 1972).

Cognitive disintegration may foster a misdiagnosis of a mental disorder, because individuals may present chaotic thinking, assaultive behavior, and an inability to be in the presence of others, resulting in complete withdrawal. Individuals with mental retardation are often misdiagnosed as suffering from atypical psychosis or schizophrenia because they cannot cope with stress in more acceptable ways. When antipsychotic drugs are prescribed under these circumstances, they may induce behaviors resulting in the further misdiagnosis of mental health symptoms.

Baseline Exaggeration

Baseline exaggeration is an increase in severity of preexisting maladaptive behavior due to periods of stress. In a person with mental retardation, a diagnostician may overlook symptoms of a mental disorder, because the symptoms exist to a lesser degree at the person's baseline level of functioning. However, the increase in severity may very well be an indication of a mental disorder.

As Sovner indicated, it is important to note that the diagnosis of a mental disorder cannot be based solely on the presence of aberrant or maladaptive behaviors. Although symptoms of mental illness are often manifested in maladaptive behaviors, a distinction exists between mental illness and behavioral problems.

Skill Development and Behavior Problems

Behavioral problems or maladaptive behaviors can occur as a result of limitations in an individual's skill development without underlying psychopathology (i.e., symptoms of mental illness). For example, physical discomfort in a nonverbal individual can result in aberrant behavior. In this case, the behavior is eliminated once the cause of the discomfort is resolved. In this example, the cause of aberrant behavior is unrelated to mental illness.

Although maladaptive behavior may not indicate the existence of a mental disorder, symptoms of mental illness are often expressed through maladaptive behaviors. For example, Dosen (1989) found psychopathology expressed through maladaptive behaviors (i.e., aggression and/or self-injury) in 100% of the cases he studied who were diagnosed with depression (described earlier). In these cases the behaviors were presumed by Dosen to be an expression of symptoms of mental illness.

The process of differentiating between a behavior disorder (i.e., the use of inappropriate behaviors to express needs or emotions) and a mental disorder (i.e., the use of inappropriate behavior as a symptom of a mental illness as defined in the *Diagnostic and Statistical Manual of Mental Disorders* [American Psychiatric Association, 1994; DSM-IV]) is often complex (Jacobson, 1990; Reiss, 1994). As a result, the accurate interpretation of aberrant behaviors and other symptoms of mental illness in people with mental retardation require the integration of both psychiatric and behavioral observation methods (Evangelista, 1988; Sovner, 1986). Singh, Sood, Somenkler, and Ellis (1998) state that "The emphasis is on the comprehensive assessment of an individual's behavior based on family history, self and informant clinical interviews, rating scales, direct observation, and an experimental analysis of target behaviors. The model provides a basis for making differential diagnoses in terms of related psychiatric disorders and behavior problems" (p. 419).

Diagnosis Instruments

The diagnosis of mental illness in people also diagnosed with mental retardation requires a modification in traditional diagnostic methods (Reiss, 1982; Sovner, 1986). As part of the strategy to adapt diagnostic methods, diagnostic screening tools have been developed to provide an inventory of observed symptoms of mental illness. Three examples of diagnostic inventories often used are the Aberrant *Behavior Checklist (ABC)* (Aman & Singh, 1986), the *Reiss Screen for Maladaptive Behaviors* (Reiss, 1986), and the *Psychopathology Instrument for Mentally Retarded Adults (PIMRA)* (Matson, 1988).

Aberrant Behavior Checklist

The *ABC* (Aman & Singh, 1986) is a 58-item informant checklist that was developed with attention to psychometric characteristics. It is divided into five subscales: (a) irritability, agitation, crying; (b) lethargy, social withdrawal; (c) stereo-typic behavior; (d) hyperactivity and noncompliance; and (e) excessive speech. The scale was originally developed to assist in the diagnosis of institutionalized patients with at least moderate levels of retardation.

Reiss Screen for Maladaptive Behaviors

The *Reiss Screen for Maladaptive Behaviors* (Reiss, 1986) is a 36-item caregiver assessment using a three-point rating scale. The *Reiss Screen* helps the diagnostician establish a mental health diagnosis when the service recipient cannot report his or her own symptoms through the gathering of vital information. There are eight factor scores related to the diagnosis of a disorder. Family members and caregivers are asked to complete the instrument and identify presenting problems within each factor from a menu of options. The development of the *Reiss Screen* is one example of increased reliance on caregivers, a development that plays an important role in efforts to improve diagnostic accuracy for people with mental retardation (Silka & Hauser, 1997).

Psychopathology Instrument for Mentally Retarded Adults

The *PIMRA* (Matson, 1988) has two parts, an informant version and a self-report. Both are recommended for use with adults with all levels of mental retardation (Hurley & Sovner, 1992). It was the first inventory to highlight the existence of depression in people with developmental disabilities. The inventory consists of 56 items and the rater answers either yes or no. The items are based on *DSM-IV* (1994) criteria in eight scales: schizophrenia, affective disorders, anxiety disorder, psychosexual disorder, adjustment disorder, somataform disorder, personality disorder, and inappropriate adjustment. It is recommended that four to seven symptoms be present to verify a specific diagnostic category.

"Mental Retardation Equivalents"

The *ABC, Reiss Screen,* and *PIMRA* are examples of the use of screening instruments designed to evoke "mental retardation equivalents" for *DSM-IV* (1994) symptoms of mental disorders (Sovner & Hurley, 1983). The use of mental health equivalents generates behavioral manifestations of symptoms found in the *DSM-IV,* such as substituting loss of appetite for a stated feeling of depressed mood (Hurley, 1996). The use of diagnostic equivalents compensates for limits in verbal ability and in self-expression often found in people with mental retardation. This helps diagnosticians differentiate between behavioral difficulties and symptoms of mental illness.

To summarize, experts believe that to interpret maladaptive behaviors with accuracy, a comprehensive examination should be conducted that takes into account both diagnostic criteria and data collection protocols based on diagnostic equivalents of symptoms of mental illness found in the *DSM-IV* (1994; Hurley, 1996; Silka & Hauser, 1997). As a result, Hurley and others point out that a mental health evaluation of people with mental retardation requires specialized training for diagnosticians. Needed resources are not always available.

Training and Resources in the Mental Health Care of People With Developmental Disabilities and Behavioral Health Care Needs

The training needs of community practitioners have long been identified as an issue affecting the quality of care people with mental retardation and developmental disabilities may receive (Szymanski & Grossman, 1984). In spite of advances in diagnostic procedures, there remains a tendency to overlook a diagnosis of a mental illness in people with mental retardation. Many observers attribute this failure to inadequate training (Hurley, 1996; Marcos, Gil, & Vazquez, 1986; Reiss, 1994; Sovner, 1986). The study of mental retardation is not part of the curriculum in 75% of the clinical psychology programs in the country (Nezu, Nezu, & Gil-Weiss, 1992). In addition, few psychiatric residency programs offer specialty training in mental retardation (Szymanski, Madow, Mallory, Menolascino, & Eidelman, 1991). In addition to training, a comprehensive evaluation requires resources, time, and collaboration between caregivers and professionals (Silka & Hauser, 1997; Sovner, Hurley, Beasley, & Silka, 1995).

Coordinated Service Delivery

There appears to be consensus among mental health policy advocates that a coordinated service structure can help alleviate the service fragmentation and associated difficulties that often occur in treating individuals with multiple service needs (Rochefort, 1993).

Four Themes of Goals of Care Systems

Four common themes emerge to describe the central goals of coordinated care systems. The four themes (as described by Kline, Harris, Bebouts, & Drake, 1993) regarding the treatment of mental illness and substance disorders are integration, comprehensiveness, flexibility, and continuity. These themes are applied below to the coordinated service needs of people with developmental disabilities and behavioral health care needs.

Integration

Services provided for people with dual diagnosis, whether on a systems level (i.e., linkage), program level (i.e., integrated), or individual level (i.e., case management), must develop a framework to integrate behavioral and mental health treatment with developmental disability or mental retardation habilitation. Coordination integrates expertise from the behavioral health and developmental disabilities service systems to provide appropriate day and residential services in addition to outpatient and inpatient mental health care.

Comprehensiveness

No one model can serve the needs of all people with dual diagnosis, and even programs targeted to serve people with developmental disabilities and behavioral health care needs must be able to treat patients with a variety of clinical presentations and levels of ability. People with developmental disabilities and behavioral health care needs require comprehensive assessments to determine specific diagnoses and levels of severity associated with rehabilitative and behavioral health care needs (Sovner, 1986). In addition, the coordinated system should include program elements to address care recipient needs at differing phases of illness and different levels of disability.

Flexibility

To address the unique needs of people with developmental disabilities and behavioral health care needs, all services and programs must be as flexible as possible in modifying traditional treatment techniques, whether for mental retardation or for mental illness. Such flexibility may include increased time and resources for appropriate diagnosis and treatment planning, emergency respite beds to assist with community transitions, planned respite to assist family caregivers, and so forth.

Continuity

Successful treatment of people with developmental disabilities and behavioral health care needs requires continuity. Longitudinally, programs treating people with developmental disabilities and behavioral health care needs must take into account changing needs and symptoms, difficulty in expressing needs, complications associated with the propensity for aberrant behaviors, and the long-term course of treatment. Across systems, people with developmental disabilities and behavioral health care needs are commonly served through multiple systems in a number of contexts, and collaboration is usually necessary to maintain a continuous focus among service providers.

Coordinated service structures are developed to improve treatment outcomes with a service structure that emphasizes a team approach through coordination, collaboration, and communication (Beasley, 1997). Most models encourage active participation in treatment planning by all members of the system; some offer respite and relief to caregivers and emergency housing for hospital diversion.

Three Alternative Strategies

Here we present three alternative strategies for coordinating care, drawing on related literature regarding mental health care for individuals without mental retardation who have severe mental health problems and/or multiple service needs. Options include case management, integrated service delivery, and a service linkage approach to coordinated service systems (Kline, Harris, Bebouts, & Drake, 1993). There is no consensus regarding which prototype of coordinated care is most effective. The different approaches to coordinating services are not mutually exclusive (Rochefort, 1993). The three major prototypes of coordinated service systems are described below.

Traditional Case Management

The first prototype, which remains the dominant one used to coordinate service delivery in the community mental health system, is the traditional case management approach. Care is provided as a result of consumer demand, and all linkages are fostered on behalf of individual care recipients. This approach offers maximum client choice of services, presuming that services in the system are accessible. The success of the traditional case management approach depends on the skills of the case manager, as well as the individual expertise of available providers. Large caseloads, lack of adequate training, and frequent turnover may create barriers to a case manager's ability to effectively coordinate individualized services (Rochefort, 1993).

Integrated Services

Integrated service systems provide multidisciplinary coordinated services under one administrative system. A team of providers, including a psychiatrist, a nurse, a social worker, and paraprofessional direct-care staff member, collaborates to address the total care needs of the dually diagnosed individual and, when applicable, the needs of family caregivers. Total care includes all needed services, such as outreach, housing support, medication supervision, crisis intervention, therapy, counseling, vocational support, recreational support, and so forth. This approach guarantees that the service team coordinates services. Some argue that the integrated approach to mental health care limits service options for individual users and restricts their ability to access generic services when they could benefit from this option (Kline, Harris, Bebouts, & Drake, 1993). For people with mental retardation, for example, many advocates do not support the use of an integrated model of service delivery, because it creates a parallel and segregated mental health system for people with mental retardation, and this can be costly due in part to administrative duplication (Rochefort, 1993). In addition, the distinct system may not be appropriate for everyone with mental retardation who has mental illness. Therefore the system may not be able to meet the needs of all people under the general category of "dual diagnosis," creating additional service gaps (Szymanski, 1977).

Service Linkage Prototype

In this approach to coordinated delivery, service linkage teams promote interdisciplinary treatment planning and service delivery, while clarifying each person's role in the ongoing provision of mental health care (Beasley & Kroll, 1999). A service linkage team's aim is to help service users, caregivers, and providers compensate for fragmentation and gaps found in the service system. Supports provided by service linkage teams may include consultation, training, and service planning and development. In some cases additional services are provided to fill in existing service gaps. For the most part, however, the service linkage team is not a primary service provider. Rather, like the traditional case management method, the mission of the service linkage team is to facilitate coordination and improvement in existing services. Therefore, most of the services used in the context of a service linkage system are independent of one another both administratively and fiscally. Unlike traditional case management, the service linkage approach has affiliation agreements that are negotiated administratively between systems rather than based on individual service needs alone. Like the other two approaches to coordination just outlined, service linkage has some difficulties associated with the approach.

Coordinated Service Systems for People With Developmental Disabilities and Behavioral Health Care Needs

For the most part, the community service system has not adequately addressed the needs of people with developmental disabilities and behavioral health care needs (Fletcher, 1993). The problems associated with poor mental health service delivery were described in two separate reports of the President's Committee on Mental Retardation (President's Commission on Mental Health, 1978, 1988). The reports described a fragmented service delivery system in which people with developmental disabilities and behavioral health care needs are frequently falling through the cracks.

According to the 1978 report (President's Commission on Mental Health), people with developmental disabilities and behavioral health care needs were "neglected by both the mental health and mental retardation service systems" (p. 2007). The presence of separate service structures had important consequences for people with developmental disabilities and behavioral health care needs who need both types of services (Reiss, 1994). In many cases there was a lack of clearly articulated policy for addressing the specific needs of individuals with dual diagnosis (Fletcher, 1993). The result has been a diffusion of responsibility and a lack of services. When services were provided, often both services and supports were fragmented (Boggs, 1988; Leismer, 1989).

Ten years later, the 1988 President's Commission report was unable to cite significant improvements in service delivery. Robert Gettings recommended four basic strategies to be pursued simultaneously to foster change in the system. He recommended that local communities and state systems:

1. Foster interagency collaboration and cooperation at the administrative and public policy levels. Gettings recommended that administrators operating separate mental health and mental retardation state governmental agencies formally arrange for information and resource sharing on behalf of individuals with dual diagnosis.

2. Assure that professionals are encouraged to collaborate across disciplines and participate in joint forums for service and treatment planning.

3. Develop an agreed-upon common diagnostic language and protocols for the care and treatment of individuals with developmental disabilities and behavioral health care needs to avoid having individuals bouncing back and forth between the mental health and retardation systems, with neither system having the resources or responsibility to meet the individual's needs.

4. Determine the efficacy of existing and newly formulated methods of mental health service delivery to people with developmental disabilities and behavioral health care needs.

Gettings (1988) suggested that top management at the state and local levels be fully committed to an effort to coordinate mental health and mental retardation services on behalf of individuals requiring a dual system of service use. Gettings recommended that local committees made up of stakeholders in the existing community system assess the current state of service delivery and determine the need for resources and shifts in the service structure. He suggested that obstacles to effective service delivery be identified through these forums and that collaborative efforts across service systems take place to remove the obstacles. The consensus from the President's Commission (1988) was that in some cases a separate system to care for people with dual diagnosis be developed, but for the most part what was needed was a clear commitment to serving these individuals by the existing system.

A Review of Some Coordinated Service Models for People With Developmental Disabilities and Behavioral Health Care Needs

A general description of coordinated service models is drawn from a literature review of model programs listed in Table 6.1. The majority of the coordinated ser-

TABLE 6.1
Programs Designed to Coordinate Mental Health Care for
People With Developmental Disabilities

Author(s), Year	Program Name
Beasley, Kroll, & Sovner, 1992	START clinical and respite services
Casner, 1996	Austin-Travis County MHMR Center
Colond & Weisler, 1995	Cambridge Minnesota Regional Support Team
Davidson, Cain, Sloane-Reeves, Giesow, Quijano, Heyningen, & Shoham, 1995	The Rochester Crisis Intervention Program
Menolascino, 1989	Encor
Middelhoff, 1996	The Netherlands model
Patterson, Higgins, & Dyck, 1995	Case Management Mental Health Network
Rambow & Arnold, 1996	The Alaska cross systems approach
Resources for Community Living, 1993	Vermont Crisis Intervention Services
Rudolph, Lakin, Oslund, & Larson, 1998	The Minnesota Special Services Program
Woodward, 1993	Interface

vice models designed to meet the needs of people with developmental disabilities and behavioral health care needs describe a service linkage philosophy of coordinated service delivery. All of the model programs also provide specialized services to enhance the system or fill in service gaps. (In a model restricted to service linkage alone, services would not be provided by the service linkage team.) Differences in resources and funding resulted in differences in the amount and type of services provided. The common and prevailing emphasis in all program models found in the literature is on coordination of services through service linkage rather than the development of a segregated service system.

All model programs employ interdisciplinary service linkage teams with expertise in dual diagnosis to coordinate services. A central goal of service linkage teams is to facilitate a coordinated effort to identify individuals who may be at risk, so as to assist caregivers and service recipients develop strategies to handle difficulties should they arise. In most cases the service linkage team receives direct funding from a state agency (usually the department of mental retardation or the department of mental health), and no service fees are charged (Beasley, Kroll, & Sovner, 1992). Most service linkage models provide both emergency support and consultation services.

In most cases services are designed to support the existing system made up of representatives from both the mental retardation and mental health service systems. Day, residential, and family support services are usually provided by the mental retardation system; psychiatric inpatient, outpatient, and emergency services are most often provided by the mental health system. The service linkage team may provide training, assistance with treatment planning, and forums for communication and collaboration, to foster a coordinated service structure. In addition, service linkage teams often provide emergency services, including 24-hour crisis evaluation services and community crisis beds.

A primary goal of service linkage teams for people with developmental disabilities and behavioral health care needs is to prevent the use of emergency mental health and psychiatric inpatient service whenever possible (Beasley, Kroll, & Sovner, 1992). Individuals in crisis may need temporary housing to ride out a difficult episode. In most cases resources made available through the service linkage team fill in service gaps. As a result, most service linkage teams provide emergency consultation and direct support services to enhance the system when needed; that is, 24-hour crisis support, psychiatry and emergency respite as an alternative to inpatient settings, or institutionalization during periods of crisis (Beasley, Kroll, & Sovner, 1992; Woodward, 1993).

The coexistence of mental retardation and mental disorders often result in behavioral crises, which the generic mental health system may have difficulty managing (Marcos, Gil, & Vazquez, 1986; Reiss, 1990; Woodward, 1993). As a result, coordinated service models need to incorporate psychiatric expertise into the interdisciplinary service linkage team and provide links with the community mental health system at large (Beasley, Kroll, & Sovner, 1992).

Consultation services often include diagnostic assistance, functional analysis, family systems consultation, and opportunities for interdisciplinary collaboration. Ongoing contact and collaboration between family caregivers (or residential providers) and professionals are essential to this process (Beasley, 1998). Planning crisis prevention and intervention strategies assist service recipients and family caregivers under stress (Beasley & Kroll, 1999). In most cases the service linkage team provides follow-up support to ensure that services remain linked and that the system is flexible in meeting the individual needs of service recipients (Rudolph, Lakin, Oslund, & Larson, 1998; Woodward, 1993).

START Model

START, an acronym for Systemic, Therapeutic, Assessment, Respite, and Treatment, has been providing clinical, emergency, and respite services to individuals since 1989. The Massachusetts Department of Mental Retardation (DMR) funds the START program to provide community-based crisis intervention and prevention service to individuals with developmental disabilities and behavioral (mental) health care needs. Figure 6.1 shows the geographic area served by the START program.

Services of Interest

To access appropriate mental health services, facilitate a coordinated service approach, and foster service linkages, START provides a number of opportunities for consultation, education, and individualized treatment planning.

In addition to five master's-level START clinicians, the consulting team is made up of two part-time psychiatrists, a neuropsychologist, a neurologist, a nurse practitioner, a forensic psychologist, a behavioral psychologist, a program development specialist, and a family systems advocacy specialist. All consultants have expertise in both developmental disabilities and behavioral health care. The consultants are also active members of the START team and meet weekly as part of an interdisciplinary team for case review with clinicians in addition to providing professional consultation.

In addition to consultation and training, START provides services to coordi-

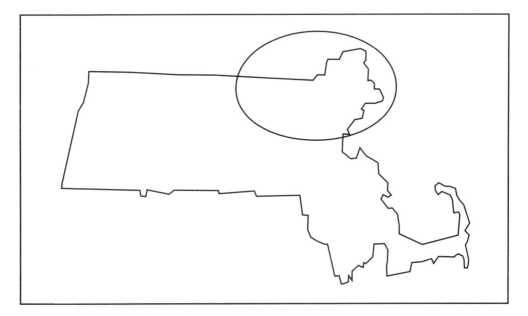

Figure 6.1. Geographic area of START services.

nate care and fill in service gaps. The services include collaborative contacts, after-hour contacts, emergency team meetings, planned respite, and emergency respite services.

Collaborative Contacts

Collaborative contacts comprise crisis prevention planning meetings, consultation visits, treatment planning meetings, and follow-up meetings.

START clinicians are required to facilitate individual crisis prevention planning meetings at least once a year. Whenever possible, the START clinician, the service user, members of the mental health service team (i.e., the outpatient therapist, a representative from the mental health crisis team, the psychiatrist), members of the mental retardation service team (i.e., the service coordinator, residential and day program providers), and the individual's informal or social supports (family members, friends, and other interested parties) meet to develop a plan to assist the individual and his or her caregivers during crises. START clinicians are also required to maintain ongoing contact with family members and other caregivers. Follow-up meetings are scheduled to evaluate the effects of treatment strategies, update crisis prevention plans, and foster active communication among providers and with direct caregivers.

After-Hour Contacts

START provides 24-hour mobile crisis services to assist in times of crisis. After regular office hours (from 5:00 P.M. to 9:00 A.M., Monday to Friday and all weekend hours), START clinicians rotate on-call responsibilities and are available to provide assistance to families, DMR, psychiatric prescreening teams, and residential providers 24 hours a day, 7 days a week. Crisis contacts may be phone calls made after hours to assist during a crisis. In addition, clinicians may provide mobile evaluation services and help a mental health crisis team determine whether or not a psychiatric inpatient admission is needed, locate an available inpatient bed, or prescreen the individual for an emergency respite admission.

Emergency Meetings

Emergency meetings are team meetings facilitated by START clinicians on a psychiatric inpatient unit or at the emergency respite facility following an admission. The meetings are scheduled within 24 hours of the admission or the next business day whenever possible. The purpose of the meeting is to allow the START clinician and other members of the team to provide information to the inpatient unit, to assist with treatment and disposition planning. Family members and residential providers are strongly encouraged to participate in the meeting. In addition, the START clinician attempts to facilitate phone contact between the individual's outpatient and inpatient psychiatrists and encourages ongoing contact between the family and residential provider throughout the admission. Whenever possible, a discharge-planning meeting is also scheduled to ensure a smooth transition back home.

The START respite facility is staffed with a full-time director, a weekend co-ordinator, direct care specialists, and awake overnight staff. The staffing pattern is three staff members to four "guests" during "awake hours" (8:00 A.M. to 10:00 P.M.) and two staff members to four guests during "sleep hours" (10:00 P.M. to 8:00 A.M.). However, one-to-one staffing is provided as needed. All guests at the respite center have private bedrooms, and one bedroom has a private bath. The center is divided into two wings, so those individuals who have more severe diffi-culties do not disturb or become disturbed by other guests. Additional facility-based emergency respite is provided by independent affiliates of START. They maintain the same staff-to-guest ratio, and work closely with START personnel.

Planned Respite

Two of the beds in the four-bed respite facility are designated as "planned respite beds." Planned respite beds at START are intended to serve individuals who have not been able to use respite in more traditional settings due to their ongoing men-tal health and/or behavioral issues. Families participating in the program must be approved by DMR as eligible for these services, but, once approved, they sched-ule visits as needed (when available).

Planned respite visits are provided to any START service recipient and are not restricted to people living with their families. An individual can visit respite for dinner, a recreational activity, or to just "check in" for a few hours. Some families visit respite with the guest to become familiar with the facility and the staff prior to scheduling an overnight bed.

Emergency Respite Services

Emergency respite services are provided at the START respite facility. Two beds in the four-bed respite facility operated by START are designated for emergency respite purposes. Unlike planned respite, which is offered only to families, all START service recipients can access emergency respite as needed pending the ap-proval of DMR. Emergency respite is designed to provide out-of-home housing and services to individuals who for a short period of time (suggested 30 or fewer days) cannot be managed at home or their residential program. Additional emer-gency respite services are purchased on an as-needed basis from START affiliates. When needed, emergency respite services were subcontracted by START with funds provided in the DMR-funded contract for the first 5 years of operation. In Year 6 the funds were removed from the START contract and services were pur-chased directly by DMR following a START request.

Psychiatric Inpatient Services

Community mental health hospitals and general community hospitals provide psychiatric inpatient mental health services. Inpatient psychiatric services are expected to be very short term (7 or fewer days). Inpatient psychiatric services are primarily provided by three hospitals in the region. The hospitals have affiliation agreements to coordinate services with START and DMR representatives. The affiliation agreements are with the hospitals with a history of providing the bulk of the inpatient services to people with MR in the region. However, other hospitals also provide some psychiatric inpatient services. START clinicians offer the same services at these times.

To access needed services, START relies upon the use of affiliation agreements and linkages with the mental retardation service system, the mental health service system, and the individual's natural support system. A diagram of the START model is provided in Table 6.2 below.

Difficulties Associated With the Service Linkage Approach to Coordinated Care

As the START system evolved over time, the service linkage approach was weak in providing services to some individuals and it became clear that additional service development was needed. This was not an unusual finding. In describing attempts to coordinate services for youth employment programs Levin and Ferman (1985) delineated three organizational issues that also affected the coordination of services on behalf of individuals with developmental disabilities and behavioral health care needs. Three difficulties associated with a coordinated service approach that primarily employs service linkage are resource scarcity, communications limitations, and organizational barriers.

Limited Resources

A service linkage approach assumes that most services are present and in suitable supply. Considering the multiple service needs of people with developmental disabilities and behavioral health care needs, availability and distribution were found to be just as serious problems as fragmentation of the service system. A good example of this is outpatient services. Many mental health clinics offer outpatient services to people with developmental disabilities as a result of a service linkage agreement, but the demand for trained personnel often exceeds the supply (Reiss, 1994). We found this to be the case in some parts of the northeast region.

Communication Limitations

A service linkage approach to coordinated service delivery requires a sophisticated tracking system to stay on top of an individual's multiple service needs. Resource availability needs to be monitored to facilitate the referral and placement process. Ongoing data collection is also needed to ensure the accountability of members

TABLE 6.2
The START Model

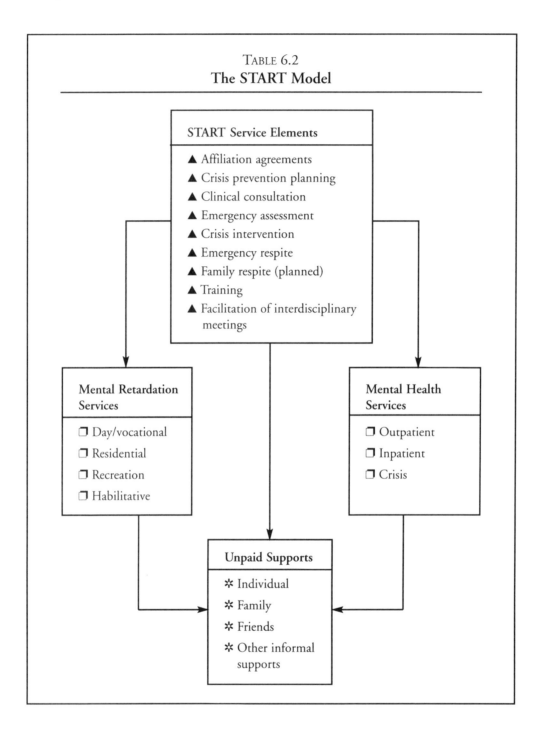

START Service Elements

▲ Affiliation agreements
▲ Crisis prevention planning
▲ Clinical consultation
▲ Emergency assessment
▲ Crisis intervention
▲ Emergency respite
▲ Family respite (planned)
▲ Training
▲ Facilitation of interdisciplinary
   meetings

**Mental Retardation
Services**

❐ Day/vocational
❐ Residential
❐ Recreation
❐ Habilitative

**Mental Health
Services**

❐ Outpatient
❐ Inpatient
❐ Crisis

Unpaid Supports

✳ Individual
✳ Family
✳ Friends
✳ Other informal
   supports

of the service system. Due to the multiple services and systems involved in some cases, this can be a complex and cumbersome process. While many individuals referred to START were successfully treated with the limited resources made available by the START team, some individuals with more complex clinical presentations were not able to benefit from generic outpatient and inpatient mental health services. Generic service providers were unable to meet the ongoing communication needs for some individuals. This resulted in ineffective services and frustration for service providers and service recipients. Some individuals placed too many communication demands on a generic system unaccustomed to meeting such demands. As a result, in some cases education and consultation were not enough to maintain constructive linkages.

Organizational Barriers

Bridging the gaps in a service delivery system made up of different organizational structures, reporting requirements, funding sources, and priorities is a complex undertaking in practice. Total cooperation among service systems is at best an uncertainty. Differing interests may create organizational conflicts that interfere with cross-systems coordination and collaboration. For example, the clinical team may advocate for a hospital stay to meet its primary goal of advocating for treatment, and the hospital may agree in meeting its primary goal to treat people with developmental disabilities and behavioral health care needs. However, these are not the only factors affecting hospital care. The generic psychiatric inpatient unit may require short lengths of stay to meet requirements of its funding source (the insurance company). In most cases the generic criteria established for treatment and discharge planning may meet the needs of an individual with developmental disabilities. But in many cases the coexistence of an acute mental health episode and developmental disabilities may require more time than a generic inpatient unit is allowed to provide. In this case the interests of the individual service user may be overshadowed by conflicting goals in a service system where an essential element is not designed to meet the needs of individuals with developmental disabilities — in spite of linkages.

In some cases service linkages alone did not meet the needs of all individuals with developmental disabilities and behavioral health care needs. As a result, both START and the community mental health system developed some specialized services.

The Development of Specialized Services

In 1989 the initial START program was funded as a four-bed respite center with a small crisis and consultation team. At that time there were no linkages to outpatient mental health services, inpatient mental health services, day treatment, day services, other respite resources, or generic community emergency mental health services. Community education and access to services along with the development of affiliations and links with existing services was our primary mission in filling the gaps in the service delivery system. As a result developing service linkages and improving systems of communication among service providers were the focus of START for the first 3 to 4 years of operation.

Over the years the START model and service philosophy evolved from an emphasis on access to services through a linkage approach to the provision of some "specialized" services. We learned that although many individuals could successfully access generic services with support, training, and education, other individuals with more severe and persistent needs required a level of experience and expertise available only through the development of specialized services. Named after our founding medical director, the late Dr. Robert Sovner, the Robert D. Sovner Behavioral Resource Center expanded in 1997 and now provides a comprehensive array of outpatient mental health services in addition to those provided in the original START model. Table 6.3 provides a comparison between the original START model with the current START/Sovner Center model. The primary difference is that in addition to accessing generic community mental health services, service users can also access specialized outpatient and inpatient mental health services designed specifically for people dually diagnosed with developmental disabilities and mental illness. Although not noted in the table, START continues to provide ongoing consultation and training. These are considered essential services.

In addition to the outpatient clinic services provided at the Sovner Center, there are currently three community psychiatric inpatient providers in Massachusetts designed to provide services specifically to individuals with developmental

TABLE 6.3
START Service Development, 1989–1999

Service	START		The START/Sovner Center	
	Linkages with generic services	Specialized services	Linkages with generic services	Specialized services
Respite	•	•	•	•
Psychiatry	•		•	•
Therapy	•		•	•
Crisis services	•	•	•	•
Day treatment			•	•
Inpatient psychiatric services	•		•	•

disabilities. All of the new services are paid through individual insurance with a small financial commitment on the part of the DMR. Therefore, the use of these services largely depends on the needs and resources of the individual service user.

START Service Population

Since its inception, START collected data regarding demographic and clinical information and START-related service use. Some data of interest are presented below.

A frequency distribution of demographic information regarding the individuals referred to START between 1989 and 1999 is outlined in Table 6.4. It is important to note that many individuals referred to START (40%) live with either family caregivers or other nonpaid supports. This finding emphasizes the need for family-professional collaboration (Beasley, 1998). In addition, it is important to

TABLE 6.4
Frequency Distribution of START Referrals, 1989–1999

Demographic	Frequency (%)
Living situation	
Residential	60.0
Live at family home	40.0
Gender	
Male	56.0
Female	44.0
Level of mental retardation	
Borderline	5.6
Mild	63.7
Moderate	19.9
Profound	9.4
Severe	1.4
Age (at time of referral)	
Under 22	6.0
22–65	67.0
Over 65	27.0
Has a diagnosed mental illness (at referral)	
Yes	56.0
No	44.0

note that START serves a significant number of individuals ages 65 and older. This finding may indicate that additional services to address clinical issues associated with aging are needed. Finally, it is important to note that only slightly more than half (56%) of the individuals referred to START for services have a diagnosed mental illness at the time of referral. This result may indicate that psychiatric disorders in individuals with developmental disabilities are underdiagnosed. This finding also emphasizes the fact that behavioral issues for people with developmental disabilities may not always be indicative of a mental illness.

Service Use

The general use of emergency, planned, and psychiatric inpatient services between 1989 and 1999 is summarized in Table 6.5. Overall, a total of 1,223 individuals with developmental disabilities and behavioral health care needs have been referred to START for services since 1989. On average START received 125 new referrals each year. With regard to planned respite, START received a total of 2,149 admissions between 1989 and 1998, with an average of 170 admissions each year. In addition, there was a total of 1,575 dinner visits to respite with an average of 193 dinner visits each year. Finally, there was a total of 681 admissions to emergency respite beds over the 10-year service period, with an average of 45 admissions per year into the two emergency respite beds.

Of interest is the average length of out-of-home respite stays and psychiatric inpatient admissions for individuals served through the START system (see Table 6.6). Planned respite stays were brief and lasted an average of approximately 2 days per admission over the 10-year service period. With regard to emergency respite admissions (with a maximum length of stay of 30 days), the average admission was far below the maximum allowed for an average of about 10 days per

TABLE 6.5
START Respite and Inpatient Use, 1989–1998

Service Type	Total (1989–1998)	M (per year)
Referrals for all Sovner Center services (number of individuals)	1,223	125
Planned respite (number of admissions)	2,149	170
Dinner visits (number of visits)	1,575	193
Emergency respite (number of admissions)	681	45

TABLE 6.6
START Average Length of Respite and Inpatient Stays, 1989–1999

Service Type	Average Length Stay (in days)
Planned respite	2.30
Emergency respite	9.63
Psychiatric inpatient	12.70

admission. Psychiatric inpatient admissions were slightly longer than emergency respite admissions, with an average length of stay of approximately 13 days per admission.

Table 6.7 outlines the average individual rate of emergency respite and psychiatric inpatient use by individuals in the START population between 1989 and 1999. The majority of individuals who used acute care beds in the community used them only once in a given year. On average, 70% of the population who used emergency respite had one admission in any given service year; 78% of the population who used psychiatric inpatient services had only one admission in the course of 1 service year.

Between 1989 and 1999, an average of 20% of those individuals who used emergency respite used them between two and three times in 1 year. With regard to inpatient psychiatric service users, an average of 14% had between two and three psychiatric admissions in a 1-year service period.

TABLE 6.7
START Average Annual Frequency of Individual Emergency Respite and Psychiatric Inpatient Service Use, 1989–1999

Number of admissions	Emergency respite (frequency of population)	Inpatient (frequency of population)
1	70%	78%
2–3	20%	14%
4–8	10%	8%

A small number of individuals who used emergency respite or psychiatric in-patient services used them more than three times in any given service year. On av-erage, this occurred in 10% of those individuals who used emergency respite ser-vices and 8% of the individuals who used psychiatric inpatient services.

The results just reviewed point to promising outcomes associated with the START coordinated service delivery system with regard to emergency service use. However, it is important to point out that the outcomes associated with the START program cannot be definitively attributed directly to the START service model because there was no comparison group.

Conclusions

This chapter presented START, a coordinated service delivery system developed to improve services for individuals with developmental disabilities and behavioral health care needs. Although originally designed as primarily a service linkage ap-proach to coordinated care, over the past 10 years START has increased its direct service capacity through the START/Sovner Center and now offers an array of specialized mental health services. Our experience at START leads us to caution program planners against the sole reliance on service linkages. Instead we suggest that a critical analysis of the existing system and service demands take place as part of program development. However, it appears that service linkages to foster coor-dinated services is an essential step and results in improved service outcomes. Re-search is needed to determine the effectiveness of START and other like service models.

References

Aman, M. G., & Singh, N. (1986). *Abberant Behavior Checklist.* East Aurora, NY: Slosson Educational Publications.

American Psychiatric Association. (1994). *Diagnostic and statistical manual of mental disorders.* (4th ed.). Washington, DC: Author.

Beasley, J. B. (1997). The three As in policy development to promote effective mental health care for people with developmental disabilities. *The Habilita-tive Mental Health Care Newsletter, 16*(2), 31–33.

Beasley, J. B. (1998). Longterm co-resident caregiving in families and persons with a dual diagnosis (mental illness and mental retardation). *Mental Health Aspects of Developmental Disabilities, 1*(1), 10–16.

Beasley, J., & Kroll, J. (1992). Who is in crisis, the consumer or the system? *Na-tional Association for the Dually Diagnosed (NADD) Newsletter, 9*(6), 1–5.

Beasley, J. B. & Kroll, J. (1999). Family caregiving part II: Family caregiver-professional collaboration in crisis prevention and intervention. *Mental Health Aspects of Developmental Disabilities, 2*(1), 22–26.

Beasley, J. B., Kroll, J., & Sovner, R. (1992). Community-based crisis mental health services for persons with developmental disabilities: The START model. *The Habilitative Mental Health Care Newsletter, 11*(9), 55–57.

Boggs, E. M. (1988). The role of legislation. In Jack A. Stark, Frank J. Menolascino, Michael H. Albarelli, & Vincent C. Gray, Eds. *Mental Retardation and Mental Health Classification, Diagnosis, Treatment, Services* (pp. 317–325). New York: Springer-Verlag.

Borthwick, S. (1988). Maladaptive behavior among the mentally retarded: The need for reliable data. In J. Stark, F. Menolascino, M. Albarelli, & V. Gray (Eds.), *Mental retardation and mental health: Classification, diagnosis, treatment services* (pp. 30–40). New York: Springer-Verlag.

Bouras, N., Kon, Y., & Drummond, C. (1993). Medical and psychiatric needs of adults with a mental handicap. *Journal of Intellectual Disability Research, 37,* 177–182.

Bregman, J. D. (1991). Current developments in the understanding of mental retardation part II: Psychopathology. *Journal of the American Academy of Child and Adolescent Psychiatry, 30,* 861–872.

Campbell, M., & Malone, R. (1991). Mental retardation and psychiatric disorders. *Hospital and Community Psychiatry, 42,* 374–379.

Carlson, G. (1981). Mental disorders and cognitive immaturity. In R. H. Belmaker & H. M. VanPraag (Eds.), *Mania: An evolving concept* (pp. 281–289). New York: Spectrum.

Casner, J. A. (1996). The Austin community support project: A collaborative treatment program provided by Austin state school and Austin-Travis County MHMR center. *National Association of Dual Diagnosis (NADD) Newsletter, 13*(1), 1–4.

Colond, J. S., & Weisler, N. A. (1995). Preventing restrictive placements through community support services. *American Journal of Mental Retardation, 100,* 201–206.

Criscione, T., Kastner, T., Walsh, K., & Nathanson, R. (1993). Managed health care systems for people with mental retardation: Impact on patient utilization. *Mental Retardation, 31*(5), 297–306.

Davidson, P., Cain, N., Sloane-Reeves, J., Giesow, V., Quijano, L., Heyningen, J. V., & Shoham, I. (1995). Crisis intervention for community based individuals with developmental disabilities and behavioral and psychiatric disorders. *Mental Retardation, 33,* 21–30.

Davidson P., Cain, N., Sloane-Reeves, J., Giesow, V., Quijano, L., & Houser, K. (1996). Factors predicting re-referral following crisis intervention for community-based persons with developmental disabilities and behavioral and psychiatric disorders. *American Journal on Mental Retardation, 101*(2), 109–118.

Davidson, P., Cain, N., Sloane-Reeves, J., VanSpeybroeck, A., Segel, J., Gutkin, J., Quijano, L., Kramer, B., Porter, B., Shoham, B., & Goldstein, E. (1994). Characteristics of community-based individuals with mental retardation and aggressive behavior disorders. *American Journal of Mental Retardation, 98,* 704–716.

Dorn, T. A., & Prout, H. T. (1993). Service delivery patterns for adults with mild mental retardation at community mental health centers. *Mental Retardation, 31,* 292–296.

Dosen, A. (1989). Community care for people with mental retardation in the Netherlands. *Australia and New Zealand Journal of Developmental Disabilities, 14,* 15–18.

Dosen, A. (1993). Diagnosis and treatment of psychiatric and behavioral disorders in mentally retarded individuals: The state of the art. *Journal of Intellectual Disability Research, 37*(1), 1–7.

Evangelista, L. A. (1988). Comprehensive management of the mentally retarded/mentally ill. In J. Stark, F. Menolascino, M. Albarelli, & V. Gray (Eds.), *Mental retardation and mental health: Classification, diagnosis, treatment services* (pp.140–146). New York: Springer-Verlag.

Fletcher, R. (1993). Mental illness and mental retardation in the United States: Policy and treatment challenges. *Journal of Intellectual Disability Research, 37*(1), 25–33.

Fletcher, R., & Poindexter, A. (1996). Current trends in mental health care for persons with mental retardation. *Journal of Rehabilitation, 62*(1), 23–25.

Fletcher, R. J., Beasley, J. B., & Jacobson, J. W. (1999). Support service systems for people with dual diagnosis. In N. Bouras (Ed.), *Psychiatric and behavioral disorders in developmental disabilities* (pp. 373–390). London: Cambridge University Press.

Gettings, R. M. (1988). Service delivery trends: A state-federal policy perspective. In J. Stark, F. Menolascino, M. Albarelli, & V. Gray (Eds.), *Mental retardation and mental health: Classification, diagnosis, treatment services* (pp. 385–393). New York: Springer-Verlag.

Ghaziuddin, M. (1988). Behavioral disorders in the mentally handicapped: The role of life events. *British Journal of Psychiatry, 152,* 683–686.

Hurley, A. D. (1996). Vocational rehabilitation approaches to support adults with mental retardation. *Habilitative Mental Healthcare Newsletter, 15*(2), 29–33.

Hurley, A. D., & Sovner, R. (1992). Inventories for evaluating psychopathology in developmentally disabled individuals. *The Habilitative Mental Healthcare Newsletter 11, 7*(8), 43–50.

Jacobson, J. W. (1982). Problem behavior and psychiatric impairment within a developmentally disabled population I: Behavior frequency. *Applied Research in Mental Retardation, 3,* 121–139.

Jacobson, J. W. (1988). Problem behavior and psychiatric impairment in a developmentally disabled population III: Psychotropic medication. *Research in Developmental Disabilities, 9,* 23–38.

Jacobson, J. W. (1990). Assessing the prevalence of psychiatric disorders in the developmentally disabled population. In E. Dibble & D. Gray (Eds.), *Assessment of persons with mental retardation living in the community* (pp. 19–70). Rockville, MD: National Institutes of Mental Health.

Jacobson, J. W. (1996). Rehabilitation services for people with mental retardation and psychiatric disabilities: Dilemmas and solutions for public policy. *Journal of Rehabilitation, 62,* 11–22.

Jacobson, J. W., & Ackerman, L. J. (1988). An appraisal of services for persons with mental retardation and psychiatric impairments. *Mental Retardation, 26,* 377–380.

Kearney, F. J., & Smull, M. W., (1992). People with mental retardation leaving mental health institutions. In J. W. Jacobson, S. N. Burchard, & P. J. Carling (Eds.), *Community living for people with developmental disabilities* (pp. 183–196). Baltimore: Johns Hopkins University Press.

Keys, V., Boroskin, A., & Ross, R. (1973). The revolving door in the MR hospital: A study of returns from leave. *Mental Retardation, 11,* 55–56.

Kline, J., Harris, M., Bebouts, R., & Drake, R. (1993). Contrasting integrated and linkages models of treatment for homeless dually diagnosed adults. *New Directions for Mental Health Services, 50,* 95–107.

Lakin, K. C., Burwell, B. O., Hayden, M. F., & Jackson, N. E. (1992). An independent assessment of the Minnesota home and community-based service waiver program (Project Rep. No. 37). Minnesota Center for Residential and Community Services.

Lakin, K. C., Prouty, B., Anderson, L., & Sandin, J. (1997). Nearly 40% of state institutions have been closed. *Mental Retardation, 35,* 65.

Levin, M. A. & Ferman, B. (1985). *The Political Hand: Policy Implementation and Youth Employment Programs.* New York: Pergamon.

MARC Mental Health Committee. (1995). Dual diagnosis: Defining dynamics, determining the dimensions. *University of Ontario Clinical Bulletin of Developmental Disabilities Program 6*(4), 1–9.

Marcos, L., Gil, R., & Vasquez, K. (1986). Who will treat psychiatrically disturbed developmentally disabled patients? A healthcare nightmare. *Hospital and Community Psychiatry, 37,* 171–174.

Matson, J. L. (1983). Depression in the mentally retarded: Toward a conceptual analysis of diagnosis. *Progress in Behavior Modification, 15,* 57–79.

Matson, J. L. (1988). *The PIMRA Manual.* Orland Park, IL: International Diagnostic Systems.

McCracken, J., & Diamond, R. (1988). Bipolar disorder in mentally retarded adolescents. *Journal of the Academy of Child and Adolescent Psychiatry, 27,* 494–499.

Mechanic, D. (1989). *Mental health and social policy.* Englewood, NJ: Prentice Hall.

Mechanic, D., & Rochefort, D. (1992). A policy of inclusion for the mentally ill. *Health Affairs, 11,* 128–150.

Menolascino, F. J. (1983). Overview. In F. J. Menolascino, & B. M. McCann, (Eds.), *Mental health & mental retardation: Bridging the gap* (pp. 3–64). Baltimore: University Park Press.

Menolascino, F. J. (1989). Model services for the treatment/management of the mentally retarded–mentally ill. *Community Mental Health Journal, 25*(2), 36–41.

Menolascino, F. J., Gilson, S. F., & Levitas, A. (1986). The nature and types of mental illness in the mentally retarded. *Psychopharmacology Bulletin, 22,* 1060-1071.

Middelhoff, L. A. (1996, October). *Case management for persons with a mental handicap and behavior and mental health problems. Results of six years of practice through cooperation of different organizations in southeast Brabant. (The Netherlands).* Paper presented at region IX annual conference, American Association of Mental Retardation, Princeton, NJ.

Nezu, C. M., Nezu, A. M., & Gil-Weiss, M. J. (1992). *Psychopathology in persons with mental retardation: Clinical guidelines for assessment and treatment.* Champaign, IL: Research Press.

Patterson, M. M., Higgins, M., & Dyck, D. (1995). A collaborative approach to reduce hospitalization of developmentally disabled clients with mental illness. *Psychiatric Services, 46*(3), 243–247.

Phillips, I., & Williams, N. (1975). Psychopathology and mental retardation: A study of 100 mentally retarded children. *American Journal of Psychiatry, 132,* 139–145.

President's Commission on Mental Health. (1978). *Report of Liaison Task Panel on Mental Retardation.* Washington, DC: U.S. Printing Office.

Rambow, T. R., & Arnold, M. (1996). Individualized/homogenized/cost effective service model. *National Association of Dually Diagnosed (NADD) Newsletter, 13*(6), 1–4.

Reiss, S. (1982). Psychopathology and mental retardation: Survey of a developmental disabilities, mental health program. *Mental Retardation, 20,* 128–132.

Reiss, S. (1986). *The Reiss screen for maladaptive behavior.* Worthington, OH: International Diagnostic Systems.

Reiss, S. (1988). *The Reiss screen test manual.* Orland Park, IL: International Diagnostic Systems.

Reiss, S. (1990). Prevalence of dual diagnosis in community-based day programs in the Chicago metropolitan area. *American Journal on Mental Retardation, 94*(6), 578–585.

Reiss, S. (1994). *Handbook of challenging behavior: Mental health aspects of mental retardation.* Worthington, OH: International Diagnostic Publishing.

Reiss, S., Levitan, G. W., & McNally, R. J. (1982). Emotionally disturbed mentally retarded people: An underserved population. *American Psychologist, 37,* 361–367.

Resources for Community Living, Inc. (1993). Moretown: Vermont Crisis Network. Unpublished program description.

Rochefort, D. A. (1993). *From poorhouses to homelessness. Policy analysis and mental health care* (pp. 134–147). Westport, CT: Auburn House.

Rudolph, C., Lakin, C., Oslund, J. M., & Larson, W. (1998). Evaluation of outcomes and cost-effectiveness of a community behavioral support and crisis response demonstration project. *Mental Retardation. 36*(3), 187–197.

Silka, V., & Hauser, M. (1997). Psychiatric assessment of persons with mental retardation. *Psychiatric Annals, 27*(3), 162–169.

Singh, N. N., Sood, A., Somenkler, N., & Ellis, A. (1998). Assessment and diagnosis of mental illness in persons with mental retardation: Methods and measures. *Behavior Modification, 15*(3), 419–443.

Smull, M. W. (1988). Systems issues in meeting the mental health needs of persons with mental retardation. In J. A. Stark, F. J. Menolascino, M. H. Albarelli, & V. C. Gray (Eds.), *Mental retardation and mental health: Classification, diagnosis, treatment services* (pp. 394–398). New York: Springer-Verlag.

Sovner, R. (1986). Limiting factors in the use of DSM-III criteria with mentally ill/mentally retarded persons. *Psychopharmacology Bulletin, 22,* 1055–1059.

Sovner, R., & Hurley, A. D. (1983). Do the mentally retarded suffer from affective illness? *Archives in General Psychiatry, 40,* 61–67.

Sovner, R., & Hurley, A. D. (1990). Assessment tools which facilitate psychiatric evaluation and treatment. *The Habilitative Mental Health Care Newsletter, 9,* 91–98.

Sovner, R., Beasley, J., & Hurley, A. D. (1995). How long should a psychiatric inpatient stay be for a person with developmental disabilities? *The Habilitative Mental Health Care Newsletter, 14*(1), 1–6.

Sovner, R., Hurley, A. D., Beasley, J., & Silka, V. (1995). Commentary: Fifteen-minute medication follow-up visits. *The Habilitative Mental Health Care Newsletter, 14*(4), 63–65.

Stancliffe, R. J., Hayden, M. F., & Lakin, C. (1999). Interventions for challenging behavior in residential settings. *American Journal on Mental Retardation, 104*(4), 364–375.

Szymanski, L. (1977). Psychiatric diagnostic evaluations of MR individuals. *Journal of the American Academy of Child Psychiatry, 16,* 67–87.

Szymanski, L., & Grossman, H. (1984). Dual implications of "dual diagnosis." *Mental Retardation, 22,* 155–156.

Szymanski, L., & Tanquey, P. (1980). Training of mental health professionals in mental retardation. In L. Szymanski & P. Tanquey (Eds.), *Emotional disorders of mentally retarded persons* (pp. 19–28). Baltimore: University Park Press.

Szymanski, L., Madow, L., Mallory, G., Menolascino, F., & Eidelman, S. (1991). *Report of the Task Force on Psychiatric Services to Adult Mentally Retarded and Mentally Disabled Persons* (Task Force Rep. No. 30). Washington, DC: American Psychiatric Association.

The President's Committee on Mental Retardation (PCMR) (1988). In Jack A. Stark, Frank Menolascino, Michael H. Albarelli, & Vincent C. Gray. (Eds.) *Mental Retardation and Mental Health, Disorders of Human Learning, Behavior and Communication.* New York: Springer-Verlag.

Woodward, H. (1993). One community's response to the multi-system service needs of individuals with mental illness and developmental disabilities. *Community Mental Health Journal, 29*(4), 347–351.

PART 3

Specialized Programs for Special Populations

CHAPTER 7

The University of Iowa Outpatient Clinic and Outreach Services

David P. Wacker
Jay Harding
Wendy K. Berg
Anjali Barretto
The University of Iowa
Iowa City, Iowa

For approximately 15 years, we have routinely conducted outpatient and outreach services that have focused on developing effective reinforcement-based treatments for people with developmental disabilities who display aberrant (i.e., self-injurious, aggressive, or destructive) behavior. These services have become fully integrated into both the Iowa University Affiliated Program and the University of Iowa Department of Pediatrics. In conjunction with our long-standing inpatient program, we have developed these services in an attempt to offer a full range of services for people with diagnosed behavioral and developmental disorders.

As shown in Table 7.1, we currently provide three distinct types of services: (a) an outpatient clinic, (b) a telemedicine consultation service, and (c) an in-home outreach service. The goals and functions of each service are distinct but are connected on both conceptual and procedural levels. Conceptually, we base all of our services on the functional analysis methodology described by Iwata, Dorsey, Slifer, Bauman, and Richman (1982/1994). Thus we believe that the best way to effectively treat aberrant behavior is to understand why the behavior is occurring. In operant terms, we assess target behavior via a functional analysis to identify the variables maintaining (reinforcing) behavior. When those variables have been identified, treatment consists of two components: (a) extinction or mild punish-

TABLE 7.1

Organization of Outpatient and Outreach Services
at the University of Iowa

	Outpatient Service	Telemedicine Service	Outreach Service
Location	University Hospital School	University Hospital School	Family homes
Number	5 to 8 per week	1 to 2 per week	Up to 10 per year
Purpose	Brief functional analysis of aberrant behavior	Ongoing functional assessment and consultation	Functional analysis and long-term treatment
Funding	Fee for service (insurance)	Grant from NLM[a]	Grant from NICHD[b]

Note. [a]Moser, M. (1997). *Specialized interdisciplinary team care for children with disabilities and consultations to their community service providers.* Washington, DC: National Library of Medicine. [b]Wacker, D. P., & Berg, W. K. (1996). *Promoting stimulus generalization with young children.* Washington, DC: National Institute of Child Health and Human Development.

ment to disrupt the response-reinforcer relation and (b) differential reinforcement of an alternative response such as appropriate communication (Carr & Durand, 1985). As discussed by Durand and Carr (1985) identifying the function of aberrant behavior is a critical first step for reinforcement-based treatment because we need to "match" treatment to the function of aberrant behavior. Thus for aberrant behavior maintained by positive reinforcement in the form of parental attention, treatment might consist of planned ignoring or nonexclusionary timeout plus contingent attention for signing "Mom." However, these components would not be therapeutic for behavior maintained by negative reinforcement in the form of escape from demands. In this case, treatment might consist of guided compliance plus brief breaks for signing "please." Knowing the function of aberrant behavior is the best way to identify effective therapeutic treatment components for any given person, and thus it is the first step in our services.

This emphasis on function has required us to substantially modify the functional analysis procedures of Iwata et al. (1982/1994). For example, we needed to develop brief versions of the procedures to conform to the time constraints of outpatient clinics (Cooper et al., 1990; Northup et al., 1991) and to ask parents (rather than trained therapists) to conduct all sessions (Derby et al., 1997; Wacker et al., 1998). This use of modified functional analyses, on a procedural level, also unifies the services. Of equal importance is our focus on reinforcement-based treatment. In each service we use the results of functional analyses to develop differential reinforcement procedures. As discussed by Derby et al. (1997), our goal is to influence the manner in which care providers and their children or consumers interact. Overall, the goal is to develop reciprocal interactions that are mutually reinforcing. We initiate this process by using a functional analysis to show the care providers that their behavior is important. During a functional analysis, target behavior often changes considerably each time a given assessment condition is presented. By demonstrating this change in behavior, we also show care providers how their behavior influences the behavior of the child or consumer.

Following the completion of the functional analysis, the next step is to implement a differential reinforcement program that not only reduces aberrant behavior (via extinction or mild punishment), but also increases adaptive behavior that is pleasing (i.e., reinforcing) to the care provider. In this way we show the child or consumer that his or her behavior is important to the care provider because of its relationship to reinforcement. Over time, then, we attempt to increase the overall amount of reinforcement that both the client and the care provider receive when they interact, even when those interactions involve previously problematic contexts (e.g., low attention or demand contexts).

In the subsequent sections, a brief description of each service is followed by a summary of outcomes. We next present a detailed case example and conclude with issues and concerns confronting each service.

Outpatient Service

The Biobehavioral Outpatient Service is a tertiary-level clinic established in 1985 at University Hospital School at the University of Iowa. The service provides functional analyses of aberrant behavior and treatment recommendations for people with developmental disabilities who engage in aberrant behaviors such as self-injury and aggression. Implementation of the treatment recommendations and long-term follow-up are provided by the patient's local care providers. An interdisciplinary team that includes the services of medicine, social work, speech and language, and psychology staffs the clinic each week.

Local physicians, education staff, group home staff, and other clinics within the University of Iowa Hospitals and Clinics refer patients to the biobehavioral clinic. Self-injury and aggression are the two most common target behaviors, but we also evaluate other problem behaviors such as property destruction, noncompliance, and stereotypy. The clinic serves people of all ages, but the majority of patients are children younger than 13 years of age.

After a referral is made, descriptive and historical information is gathered from the patient's family and school or vocational providers via questionnaires and telephone contact (i.e., an antecedent-behavior-consequence interview). This information is reviewed in conjunction with the patient's medical records, and tentative hypotheses are developed regarding the function of problem behavior. The information gathered on each patient is discussed during a multidisciplinary staffing at the beginning of each clinic day. Tentative hypotheses for problem behavior are presented, and an assessment plan is developed to test the hypotheses.

Over the past year, approximately 127 patients, ranging in age from 1 to 53 years, visited the clinic from one to three times. It was the first clinic visit for 72 of these patients and was a return visit for the remaining. Of those patients attending the clinic for the first time, the majority were children between the ages of 2 and 12 years. Self-injury or aggression were listed as the primary referral issue for 78% and 75% of the cases, respectively.

In a previous analysis of our use of brief functional analyses within the outpatient clinic (Derby et al., 1992), comparable data were reported. In addition, Derby et al. (1992) reported that for those patients who displayed aberrant behavior in the clinic (63%), the most common function (48%) was negative reinforcement. Of concern, however, is that only slightly more than half of the patients referred for evaluation displayed aberrant behavior in the clinic. For these patients, a brief functional analysis was not useful in developing treatment. However, when aberrant behavior was displayed, a distinct function was identified 74% of the time.

Case Example

Abby, a 6-year-old girl who lived with her parents and sister, was referred to the Biobehavioral Outpatient Service for aggression (i.e., pulling hair, biting), tantrums, and noncompliance. Abby's diagnoses included mental retardation, cerebral palsy, a seizure disorder, and significant communication deficits. According to the questionnaire completed by Abby's classroom teacher, problem behavior was most likely to occur when Abby was required to perform a nonpreferred activity and when she was required to work alone. Based on the teacher's questionnaire and a telephone interview with Abby's parents, we hypothesized that behavior served either an escape or an attention function.

A brief functional analysis was conducted, with Abby's parents serving as the therapists throughout each condition. Biobehavioral clinic staff provided coaching to Abby's parents throughout the functional analysis conditions.

The analysis began with a free-play condition in which Abby was allowed to play with an assortment of toys while her parents provided her with noncontingent positive social attention. The purpose of the free-play condition was to provide a control condition in which none of the variables hypothesized to affect problem behavior were present. Abby was allowed to play with the toys of her choice (no demands were made), with her parents' undivided attention. As predicted, problem behavior did not occur during this condition (see Figure 7.1).

During the next condition (alone), Abby was allowed to play with the toys of her choice, but her parents left the area and Abby was required to play alone. The purpose of this condition was to determine whether the loss of parental attention would result in problem behavior. Abby continued to play with the toys without engaging in problem behavior during this condition. Next, a contingent escape condition was conducted to evaluate the role of escape from nonpreferred activities as a reinforcer for problem behavior. In this condition, Abby's parents presented Abby with a set of washcloths to fold. Each time that Abby engaged in problem behavior such as biting or screaming, the parents removed the stack of washcloths and told Abby that she could take a short break from working. Abby displayed problem behavior for 21% of the intervals during this condition. During the attention condition, Abby was given toys to play with as her parents sat across the room and talked to the clinic staff. Abby's parents ignored her unless

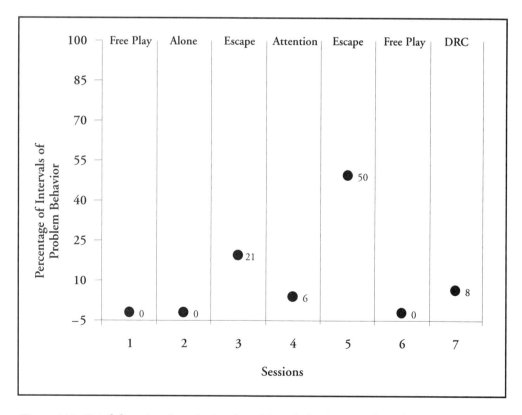

Figure 7.1. Brief functional analysis of problem behavior, conducted in an outpatient clinic. Behavior was recorded using a 6-s partial-interval system.

she engaged in problem behavior. When problem behavior occurred, her parents approached her and provided mild reprimands (e.g., "Calm down") for approximately 10 to 20 seconds. Abby engaged in low levels of problem behavior (6% of the intervals) for this condition. A second test of the contingent escape condition was conducted to form a minireversal design (i.e, quickly returning to the washcloth folding situation) as recommended by Cooper et al. (1992). Abby engaged in the highest levels of problem behavior (50% of the intervals) that were observed throughout the evaluation. A return to the free-play condition resulted in an immediate cessation of problem behavior.

The results of the functional analysis suggested that Abby was most likely to exhibit problem behavior when the behavior resulted in the removal of nonpreferred activities. In addition, the results of the functional analysis were correlated with the findings of the interviews, adding support to our conclusion that aberrant behavior was maintained by negative reinforcement. Based on these findings, a differential reinforcement of communication (DRC) treatment (Durand & Carr, 1985) was developed that required Abby to complete a small portion of the nonpreferred activity (e.g., fold one washcloth) and then sign "please" to receive a break from the activity. A practice DRC session was conducted in the clinic setting with Abby's parents presenting the nonpreferred activity to Abby and prompting Abby to sign "please" after she completed a small portion of the activity. Minimal problem behavior occurred during the DRC session even though the context (demands) had been the most problematic situation initially during the functional analysis.

Following the treatment probe, recommendations for using the treatment at home and school were discussed. Handouts that included written descriptions of the treatment were given to the parents. A follow-up phone call was arranged, and a return-as-needed clinic appointment was discussed. Routine follow-up visits are not scheduled, given both logistical constraints (families often travel more than 100 miles to attend the clinic) and constraints imposed by managed care.

Currently our clinic is doing well. Because of the number of referrals, we have recently initiated a second clinic day per week, and both days are prescheduled for almost 2 months. The greatest challenge we face is the uncertainty of managed health care, with two major issues confronting us. First, most managed care plans include special provisions for mental health services. Although many of the mental health guidelines are irrelevant for the population we serve, we often face concerns related to those guidelines. For example, the "acute" and "chronic" dimensions of behavioral disorders can be confusing to managed care agencies. Second, we often face questions regarding the feasibility or usefulness of both the assessment and the treatment procedures. Some managed care agencies, for example, still consider self-injury to be an aspect of mental retardation.

Telemedicine Service

As indicated in Table 7.1, the telemedicine service is funded by the National Library of Medicine (Moser, 1997) and not by patient fees. The goal of this service, as currently funded, is to provide a wide spectrum of clinical services via consultation or direct assessment to patients and their families and other care providers at remote, rural sites throughout Iowa. University Hospital School has a telemedicine studio, and children served by our specialists are evaluated via live, interactive audiovisual sessions. In our studio, two video monitors display the clinic staff and local staff, parents, and consumers at the remote (local) site. Throughout Iowa, studios of this type are located in most high schools, in many regional hospitals, and in a variety of educational buildings. Our current grant provides funding for a telemedicine coordinator in our hospital and in Ottumwa, Iowa, which is located in a rural area. A major goal of the project was to determine whether the consultation provided by our outpatient clinic could be conducted just as effectively, but more efficiently, via our telemedicine service.

A typical outpatient visit to University Hospital School includes evaluations by several disciplines (e.g., psychology, speech, social work, education, physical therapy), and the patient and family can expect to spend the entire day at the hospital. For people traveling long distances to bring their children for an evaluation, this is sometimes inconvenient and expensive. For example, parents may need to take time off from work and hire a babysitter for their other children. The introduction of telemedicine services has reduced these inconveniences because it provides an opportunity for a team of specialists to evaluate a child in a relatively short period of time (e.g., 30 to 60 minutes) at a location very close to the family's home.

Telemedicine services include both initial and follow-up evaluations, but the emphasis is on follow-up consultation (see Table 7.2). As in our outpatient clinic, initial evaluations focus on identifying the environmental variables maintaining problem behavior. This assessment includes both descriptive (A-B-C interview) and brief functional analyses.

When conducting initial functional analyses, we always have a local teacher or psychologist conduct the sessions with the parent. In four cases, in which we had the initial evaluation via telemedicine, the teacher or psychologist was experienced in functional analysis but wanted ongoing guidance. In these cases we met for 15 to 30 minutes prior to a 60-minute functional analysis session to discuss the assessment conditions. Following the assessment, a brief phone call was conducted as a wrap-up if needed. Three of the four functional analyses were successful in that a function for problem behavior was identified. Of interest is that two of these successful evaluations involved children who were of normal intelligence but had diagnosed behavior disorders. These results suggest that telemedicine options might

TABLE 7.2
Summary of Telemedicine Evaluations Conducted at
University Hospital School

	Initial Evaluation via Telemedicine	Follow-up Evaluation	Other Evaluations
Type	Functional analysis A-B-C assessment	Ongoing consultation	Discharge conference Short-term consultation
Referral source	School Parents or care providers Group home	Biobehavioral inpatient service Biobehavioral outpatient service	School Parents or care providers Group Home
Number (11/96– present)	4	43	20

be considered for conducting brief functional analyses and especially for children who live in remote areas or long distances from the clinic or center. In the cases of the two children just mentioned, the evaluations occurred in Des Moines, a large urban setting located more than 100 miles from our clinic. Given the initial success of these two evaluations, up to 10 more telemedicine evaluations are planned for the next school year, and all will be initial assessments involving brief functional analyses.

Follow-up evaluations consist of ongoing consultation by our clinic team after an initial evaluation has been conducted by the biobehavioral inpatient or outpatient services. We believe that these types of follow-up consultations will be the greatest advantage of telemedicine services. The initiation of reinforcement-based treatments are often challenging to local service providers and parents. Extinction bursts, satiation of reinforcers, changes in prompting strategies, and idiosyncratic influences of the local environment may all pose concerns for durable treatment. Frequent follow-up in which visual contact is made with local care providers often can address these concerns relatively quickly.

Case Example
Karl was 8 years old, lived with his parents and a younger sibling, and was diagnosed with autism and deafness. He was referred to the Biobehavioral Outpatient

Service by his family physician and his parents for an evaluation of behavioral concerns, including self-injury (e.g., head banging, eye poking), aggression (e.g., hitting others), destruction, stereotypy (e.g., key twirling), and lack of independent toy play. During an initial outpatient evaluation in our biobehavioral clinic, we conducted a brief functional analysis to identify the environmental variables maintaining Karl's problem behavior. Karl's parents conducted all sessions with assistance from clinic staff. The results of this assessment identified that Karl's aberrant behavior (e.g., self-injury) served several social functions depending on the context (e.g., to gain preferred items or to escape nonpreferred demands). In addition to self-injury, we observed that Karl wandered around the therapy room continuously and resisted his parents when they attempted to engage him in a play activity. We recommended a treatment package that included structured work and play situations, choice making, functional communication training, and extinction. This package of procedures was demonstrated by clinic staff and described in written recommendations that were subsequently sent to the family.

Given both the severity and the complexity of Karl's target behavior, we believed that it was necessary to view these recommendations as part of an ongoing assessment in the home. We scheduled routine follow-ups via the telemedicine service, with the first occurring 1 month after the clinic evaluation to determine the efficacy of our recommendations. All providers working with Karl (e.g., in-home therapist, teacher, speech therapist, family physician) were invited to attend, and all did attend at least one session. During this follow-up evaluation, Karl's parents and the in-home therapist raised concerns regarding specific situations. For example, Karl's parents reported that he was not generalizing his play skills (e.g., Karl would play with the in-home therapist but not with his parents). The in-home therapist reported that stereotypic behavior continued to occur at a high frequencies and was disruptive during work situations. To address both of these problems, we advised the family to conduct frequent preference assessments to isolate the sensory components of stereotypy (i.e., the sensory stimuli that might have functioned as reinforcers), which helped us to identify alternative reinforcers to serve as substitutes for stereotypy. We also recommended the use of an A-B-C observation system to record Karl's behaviors during the day so that, on subsequent sessions, we could initiate treatment during the most problematic times. Detailed procedures and observation forms were provided for conducting these assessments. This type of ongoing consultation, in which alternative methods of assessment and treatment were incorporated into an overall plan, was critical for monitoring ongoing behavioral progress.

To date, we have conducted eight follow-up telemedicine consultations with this family. All evaluations were attended by Karl's parents, and most also included the in-home therapist and the speech therapist. In addition, frequent phone contact occurred, and the family sent us videotapes documenting Karl's progress.

During the course of this long-term consultation, Karl displayed substantial improvement in most of his behaviors. His interactive toy play with his parents increased, and we then targeted independent toy play. His stereotypic behaviors showed a marked decrease. His aggressive behavior decreased either to zero or to very manageable levels across various settings. Because of the availability of the telemedicine service, we were able to establish and maintain a collaborative and consistent plan across both home and school.

The most pressing concern for telemedicine services is that, because of its newness, it is not covered under most mental health managed care plans. To date, all services (near Ottumwa) have been funded by the grant or, near Des Moines, by local agencies. We have waived our professional fees for all cases, as have local service providers. Our challenge is to convince managed care agencies, through education and consultation, that telemedicine is an effective and cost-efficient service.

Community Outreach Service

This service has been funded in part by the National Institute of Child Health and Human Development (Wacker & Berg, 1992a, 1996) and the National Institute on Disability and Rehabilitation Research (Wacker & Berg, 1992b). In these programs there were 94 families with young children (ages 8 months to 8 years) who have a variety of disabilities and engage in severe problem behavior (e.g., aggression, self-injury, property destruction, food refusal). All assessment and treatment procedures are conducted by the child's primary care provider (usually a parent), with a clinic therapist providing coaching during visits to the child's home or other community settings. Assessment and treatment procedures in these programs have been videotaped for subsequent data analysis.

Our outreach programs involve a multiphase model of assessment, treatment, and treatment evaluation (see Table 7.3). In Phase 1 (descriptive assessment) parents provide current information on their child's behavior across routine activities and settings. During Phase 2 (functional analysis) we conduct a functional analysis of behavior based on hypotheses generated during the descriptive assessment. In Phase 3 (treatment) parents conduct an individualized treatment program (e.g., functional communication training) that is matched to the assessment outcomes. During Phase 4 (treatment follow-up) weekly to monthly treatment probes are conducted to evaluate the effectiveness, maintenance, and/or generalization of treatment effects. Consumer satisfaction with the treatment is assessed by having the parent complete a treatment acceptability survey, *Treatment Acceptability Rating Form — Revised* (Reimers & Wacker, 1988 [*TARF-R*]).

TABLE 7.3
Outreach Assessment and Treatment Procedures

Method	Purpose
Phase 1: Descriptive Behavior record Interview Preference assessment	Identify routine events associated with problem behavior. Clarify parent concerns; generate hypotheses. Identify preferred toys and activities.
Phase 2: Functional *analysis*	Identify maintaining variables for problem behavior.

Phase 3: Treatment
Functional communication
training (FCT)
	Teach child to request reinforcement
	  appropriately; withhold reinforcement
	  for problem behavior.

Phase 4: Treatment *follow-up*	Evaluate treatment effects across time and generalization contexts.

Phase 1: Descriptive Assessment

The first step in our service is to ask parents to record their child's behavior for 1 week. The parent uses a behavior recording form to indicate the occurrence of problem behavior during 30-minute intervals throughout the day (Touchette, McDonald, & Langer, 1985). Parents also are asked to include a brief description of the activities that preceded or occurred at the same time as the problem behavior (Bijou, Peterson, & Ault, 1968). We conduct interviews to clarify the results of the behavior record and to develop preliminary hypotheses regarding the events that may be related to the child's problem behavior (O'Neill, Horner, Albin, Storey, & Sprague, 1989).

Descriptive assessments are useful as a means of formulating hypotheses with respect to variables that may be influencing the child's behavior (Harding, Wacker, Cooper, et al., 1999; Lalli & Goh, 1993). However, the complexity of events that occur in natural environments may generate multiple hypotheses (Mace & Lalli, 1991). Thus it is important to conduct an experimental analysis to identify functional relations between behavior and environmental events.

Phase 2: Functional Analysis

During the functional analysis, a series of assessment conditions are conducted in which a reinforcer is provided to the child contingent on the occurrence of problem behavior. Because we are working in the home for an extended period of time, we are able to conduct the functional analysis over several days. In most cases the analysis is completed in two to three visits to the home but, in more complex cases, may continue for several weeks. We typically conduct free play, contingent attention, contingent tangible, and contingent escape analogue conditions. In cases where an idiosyncratic variable is identified via the descriptive assessment (e.g., different patterns of responding in and out of wheelchair), we will conduct each condition in both the presence and the absence of the idiosyncratic variable to more precisely evaluate behavior.

Phase 3: Treatment

As mentioned earlier, in our outreach programs we recommend two essential elements in the treatment procedures. First, we ask the parent to provide reinforcement only for appropriate behavior. Second, we ask the parent to remove, or reduce, reinforcement for problem behavior. Of the many variations of differential reinforcement procedures used in behavioral intervention, our programs emphasize functional communication training (Carr & Durand, 1985). The goal of Functional Communication Training is to replace problem behavior with an appropriate communicative response (i.e., a mand) that serves the same function as the problem behavior. For example, if problem behavior is maintained by attention, the child is taught an appropriate way to request attention. Depending on the child's abilities, the mand may be vocal, a manual sign, a gesture, or a signal from an external device (e.g., a recorded message on a microswitch). Conversely, the parent withholds or minimizes attention for problem behavior. Thus the parent teaches the child that asking for attention appropriately is more likely to be reinforced than engaging in problem behavior.

Phase 4: Treatment Follow-up

Treatment evaluation is an important component of our outreach programs. After a treatment has been developed, we continue to make weekly visits to the child's home. During these follow-up visits, we provide coaching and feedback on treatment implementation, address questions and concerns, and assess treatment efficacy. We may also provide consultation to other community service providers who are involved with the family. The average duration of treatment follow-up across our programs has been approximately 8 months. For programs that have enabled us to maintain long-term involvement with the family (Derby et al., 1997; Wacker et al., 1998), we typically faded out scheduled visits to 1-month intervals after documenting consistent improvement in child behavior. Although our contact with the family was reduced, these monthly visits enabled us to evaluate the maintenance of treatment effects over time and to address emerging issues as the child developed.

In our most recent project (Wacker & Berg, 1996), we also assessed the generalization of in-home treatment outcomes across multiple settings in the community (e.g., school, relative's homes), care providers (e.g., teachers, in-home service providers, relatives), and tasks (e.g., daily care activities, academic tasks, play activities) that had been identified as being associated with problem behavior. This approach enabled us to address behavioral concerns across multiple contexts in a systematic fashion. In cases where treatment effects did not generalize to a satisfactory degree, we provided additional treatment recommendations and then continued to monitor the child's progress.

Summary Data

We have published a number of articles and monographs that provide outcome data for participants in our outreach programs (Derby et al., 1997; Harding, Wacker, Berg, et al., 1999; Peck et al., 1996; Wacker et al, 1998). To date, our most comprehensive discussion of outreach program results (Wacker et al., 1998) showed that the 24 children who received in-home treatment demonstrated an average decrease in aberrant behavior of 87% (range, 45% to 100%) from baseline levels. Children in this program also displayed increases in appropriate social responding to their parents. At the conclusion of the program, 20 parents completed treatment acceptability surveys. Overall treatment acceptability was rated on a scale of 1 (not at all acceptable) to 7 (highly acceptable). Average ratings were 6.35 (range, 4 to 7).

Our other outreach programs have had similar outcomes with respect to reductions in aberrant behavior and treatment acceptability. For example, using another sample of 36 children (Wacker & Berg, 1992b), aberrant behavior decreased an average of 80% following at least 2 months of treatment. Preliminary results from our most recent project (Wacker & Berg, 1996) showed that 88% of the children who received in-home treatment (n = 16) showed reductions in aberrant behavior of 80% or more from baseline levels.

Although these results are encouraging, there remains a significant percentage of children who did not display what we consider to be "successful" reductions in aberrant behavior (80% or more). For example, Wacker et al. (1998) showed that all project participants who received treatment (N = 24) displayed a substantial decrease in aberrant behavior; however, for eight of these children, the reduction was less than 80%. Although we may attribute this more modest reduction to a variety of variables, the fact remains that we must continue our efforts to provide effective and acceptable treatment options.

Case Example

Ken was 2.5 years old and was diagnosed with severe developmental delays and a seizure disorder. Ken displayed no language development. Problem behaviors included destruction of property (e.g., throwing and pulling down objects) and

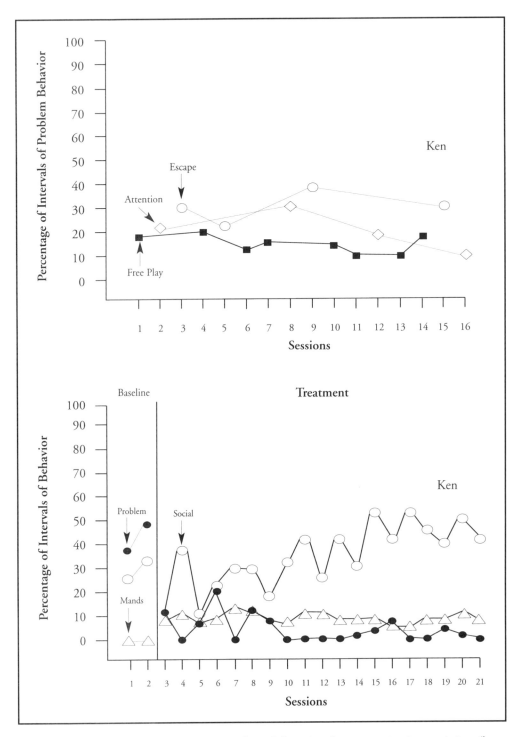

Figure 7.2. Functional analysis (top panel) and functional communication training (bottom panel) results for a participant in an outreach program. Behavior was recorded using a 6-s partial-interval system.

aggression (e.g., scratching, pulling hair). Ken's destructive behavior was so severe that his mother was forced to remove all portable items from the living room.

Ken's functional analysis consisted of three assessment conditions: free play, contingent attention for problem behavior, and contingent escape for problem behavior. The results (top panel of Figure 7.2) showed that Ken engaged in problem behavior across all three conditions, with slightly higher elevations during the contingent escape condition. Although reducing Ken's destructive behavior was a primary objective, we also wanted to increase his ability to follow directions and to engage in appropriate social interactions with his mother.

During Ken's functional communication training, his mother taught him to sit and complete simple requests (e.g., placing objects in a sorting container). If Ken completed several requests appropriately, he was given an opportunity to request a "break" by touching a sign. During his break, he was allowed to select a toy, and his mother played with him. If he engaged in problem behavior, he was immediately required to return to his work task. Thus Ken's training program consisted of multiple components. First, he was required to complete a task that was associated with problem behavior during the functional analysis. Second, he was required to communicate that he wanted a break from his task. Third, Ken's breaks always included efforts by his mother to engage him in appropriate toy play. Finally, displays of problem behavior always resulted in a return to work.

The results of Ken's treatment across 2 years of follow-up probes are shown in the bottom panel of Figure 7.2. During baseline probes, Ken displayed high levels of problem behavior and relatively low levels of appropriate social behavior (e.g., toy play, interaction with his mother). During treatment, Ken learned to follow parent directions and to mand for a break from his work task. His problem behavior decreased substantially and his appropriate social behaviors increased.

Issues and Concerns

Although the results of these programs have been encouraging, there are several issues that relate to the relative success achieved for any given child. First, it is critical to establish an active collaborative relationship with the child's care provider. If our recommendations are unacceptable to the care provider, then it is not likely that treatment will be conducted with both the frequency and the integrity needed to promote behavioral change. Second, children grow, develop new skills and interests, or experience changes in health status. Thus we must be prepared to reassess and, if needed, modify our treatment programs so that they continue to meet the child's needs. Third, a child's environment may be altered during the course of treatment. For example, many of the children in our projects experience changes in their family structure, residence location, or educational programming. For this reason, the use of telemedicine services might be a practical and useful method for augmenting these relatively more expensive in-home services.

Finally, our outreach services, like the telemedicine services, are funded entirely by grants. To date, we have been unable to secure ongoing funding from sources other than grant agencies. To be successful, we need to develop effective training procedures for early intervention and in-home service providers who are employed by schools or by programs such as the MR waiver program.

Summary

In this chapter we have provided a brief description of our services that are based in outpatient and community settings. Our outpatient clinic, like our inpatient program, is fully funded by patient fees and long-standing appropriations. These services are now considered to be "routine" in our hospital, as are procedures such as the functional analyses used in the clinic.

The telemedicine service, as the newest service, is the most tentative. However, it has been received with enthusiasm by our clinic staff, others in the hospital, and parents and local service providers. We fully expect that our telemedicine service will become an integrated component in our overall service delivery.

Our outreach service is quite simply the best of what we have to offer. The opportunity to work in a collaborative fashion with parents in their homes offers too many advantages to summarize. The outcomes associated with this service support its effectiveness. Unfortunately, unless supported by research grants or contracts, it is not viable because of expense. Although various types of in-home services are available to parents with children who have developmental and behavioral disorders, few are focused on functional approaches to assessing and treating aberrant behavior. The common objectives of our services — to evaluate the function of aberrant behavior and to develop reinforcement-based treatments — offer a type of program that is not available to most families. In our view, the type (structure) of the community-based program is not as important as a clearly focused set of objectives. When the objectives are clear, then any number of alternative structures and formats may be successful. For us, the focus on function has been the critical variable.

Author Note

This chapter was supported in part by the Iowa University Affiliated Program, the National Library of Medicine, and the National Institute of Child Health and Human Development. However, the opinions expressed do not necessarily reflect those of the funding agencies.

References

Bijou, S. W., Peterson, R. F., & Ault, M. H. (1968). A method to integrate descriptive and experimental field studies at the level of data and empirical concepts. *Journal of Applied Behavior Analysis, 1,* 175–191.

Carr, E. G., & Durand, V. M. (1985). Reducing behavior problems through functional communication training. *Journal of Applied Behavior Analysis, 18,* 111–126.

Cooper, L. J., Wacker, D. P., Sasso, G. M., Reimers, T. M., & Donn, L. (1990). Using parents as therapists to evaluate appropriate behavior of their children: Application to a tertiary diagnostic clinic. *Journal of Applied Behavior Analysis, 23,* 285–296.

Cooper, L., Wacker, D., Thursby, D., Plagmann, L., Harding, J., Millard, T., & Derby, M. (1992). Analysis of the effects of task preferences, task demands, and adult attention on child behavior in outpatient and classroom settings. *Journal of Applied Behavior Analysis, 25,* 823–840.

Derby, K. M., Wacker, D. P., Berg, W., DeRaad, A., Ulrich, S., Asmus, J., Harding, J., Prouty, A., Laffey, P., & Stoner, E. A. (1997). The long-term effects of functional communication training in home settings. *Journal of Applied Behavior Analysis, 30,* 507–531.

Derby, K. M., Wacker, D., Sasso, G., Steege, M., Northup, J., Cigrand, K., & Asmus, J. (1992). Brief functional assessment techniques to evaluate aberrant behavior in an outpatient setting: A summary of 79 cases. *Journal of Applied Behavior Analysis, 25,* 713–721.

Durand, V. M., & Carr, E. G. (1985). Self-injurious behavior: Motivating conditions and guidelines for treatment. *School Psychology Review, 14,* 171–176.

Harding, J. W., Wacker, D. P., Berg, W. K., Cooper, L. J., Asmus, J., Mlela, K., & Muller, J. (1999). An analysis of choice making in the assessment of young children with severe behavior problems. *Journal of Applied Behavior Analysis, 32,* 63–82.

Harding, J., Wacker, D. P., Cooper, L. J., Asmus, J., Jensen-Kovalan, P., & Plagmann, L. A. (1999). Combining descriptive and experimental analyses of young children with behavior problems in preschool settings. *Behavior Modification, 23,* 325–342.

Iwata, B. A., Dorsey, J. F., Sliffer, K. J., Bauman, K. E., & Richman, G. S. (1982/1994). Toward a functional analysis of self-injury. *Journal of Applied Behavior Analysis, 27,* 197–209. (Reprinted from [1982] *Analysis and Intervention in Developmental Disabilities, 2,* 3–20).

Lalli, J. S., & Goh, H. (1993). Naturalistic observations in community settings. In J. Reichle & D. Wacker (Eds.), *Communicative alternatives to challenging behavior: Integrating functional assessment and intervention strategies* (pp. 11–39). Baltimore: Paul H. Brookes.

Mace, F. C., & Lalli, J. S. (1991). Linking descriptive and experimental analyses in the treatment of bizarre speech. *Journal of Applied Behavior Analysis, 24,* 553–562.

Moser, M. (1997). *Specialized interdisciplinary team care for children with disabilities and consultations to their community service providers.* Washington, DC: National Library of Medicine.

Northup, J., Wacker, D. P., Sasso, G., Steege, M., Cigrand, K., Cook, J., & De-Raad, A. (1991). A brief functional analysis of aggressive and alternative behavior in an outclinic setting. *Journal of Applied Behavior Analysis, 24,* 509–522.

O'Neill, R. E., Horner, R. H., Albin, R. W., Storey, K., & Sprague, J. R. (1989). The functional analysis interview. In R. H. Horner, J. L. Anderson, E. G. Carr, G. Dunlap, R. L. Koegel, & W. Sailor (Eds.), *Functional analysis: A practical assessment guide* (pp. 10–23). Eugene: University of Oregon Press.

Peck, S. M., Wacker, D. P., Berg, W. K., Cooper, L. J., Brown, K. A., Richman, D., McComas, J. J., Frischmeyer, P., & Millard, T. (1996). Choice-making treatment of young children's severe behavior problems. *Journal of Applied Behavior Analysis, 29,* 263–290.

Reimers, T., & Wacker, D. (1988). Parents' ratings of the acceptability of behavioral intervention recommendations made in an outpatient clinic: A preliminary analysis of the influence of intervention effectiveness. *Behavioral Disorders, 14,* 7–15.

Touchette, P. E., MacDonald, R. F., & Langer, S. N. (1985). A scatterplot for identifying stimulus control of problem behavior. *Journal of Applied Behavior Analysis, 18,* 343–351.

Wacker, D. P., & Berg, W. K. (1992a). *Inducing reciprocal parent/child interactions.* Washington, DC: National Institute of Child Health and Human Development, U.S. Department of Health and Human Services.

Wacker, D. P., & Berg, W. K. (1992b). *Functional analysis of feeding and interaction disorders with young children who are profoundly disabled.* Washington, DC: Department of Education, National Institute on Disability and Rehabilitation Research.

Wacker, D. P., & Berg, W. K. (1996). *Promoting stimulus generalization with young children.* Washington, DC: National Institute of Child Health and Human Development, U.S. Department of Health and Human Services.

Wacker, D. P., Berg, W. K., Harding, J. W., Derby, K. M., Asmus, J. M., & Healy, A. (1998). Evaluation and long-term treatment of aberrant behavior displayed by young children with disabilities. *Journal of Developmental and Behavioral Pediatrics, 19,* 260–266.

CHAPTER 8

The Pueblo DD-MH Consortium Model of Behavioral Support and Crisis Response

Lawrence A. Velasco
Lamar Trant
Colorado Bluesky Enterprises
Pueblo, Colorado

Peter Holmes
Eastern Michigan University,
Ypsilanti, Michigan

During the 1980s health officials in Colorado actively worked to deinstitutional-ize many people with developmental disabilities who resided in the three existing state regional centers. In 1980 the population in institutions was more than 2,200, and by 1985 the population had been reduced in half (Colorado Depart-ment of Human Services, 1999). Many of these individuals received services from community-centered boards (CCBs), private nonprofit agencies that were serving about 6,000 individuals in 20 different geographic areas throughout the state. Ad-ditionally, deinstitutionalization efforts were furthered in 1985 when Colorado implemented new legislation and policies, which recognized and guaranteed full rights to all people with developmental disabilities. Thus individuals could no longer be held in institutions against their will and subsequently many individu-als elected to leave institutions and live in the surrounding areas of the state's three regional centers.

Historically, Pueblo, Colorado, served as a catchment center for developmen-

tally disabled, mentally ill, and law-breaking Colorado citizens who were returning from an institutional placement to the community. This situation was due to
the location of the Colorado State Hospital and one of the state's three regional
centers for individuals with developmental disabilities as well as several prison facilities within a 50-mile radius of Pueblo. The imminent downsizing of the area
state developmental disabilities facilities created many problems: Where should
the difficult-to-manage institutional residents live? Who should be responsible for
their care? How should local law enforcement deal with people who formerly
would have been sent to an institution? Who was going to pay for needed services
in times of limited funds?

The problems faced by service providers in Pueblo were not unique to this region (Fidura, Lindsey, & Walker, 1987). Individuals classified as dually diagnosed
(i.e., significantly subaverage intellectual functioning accompanied by a condition
of mental illness) have traditionally had a difficult time securing appropriate and
effective services (Lord & Pedlar, 1991; Menolascino, Gilson, & Levitas, 1986).
Model programs have often had limited success, unreliable support, and a premature end. Service agencies for people with developmental disabilities (DD) and
those serving mental health (MH) clients inherently mistrust one another over the
dual-diagnosis issue (Szymanski, 1987). Definitions, ownership, and solutions for
people with a dual diagnosis have continued to be a constant issue for debate and
frustration.

In 1987 representatives of Pueblo service providers in the developmental disabilities field and the mental health field met to discuss mutual problems and the
lack of trust between systems. It was evident that the region lacked comprehensive and coordinated services for people with a dual diagnosis. Mental health representatives felt that the developmental disabilities system should serve all people
with developmental disabilities. Developmental disabilities representatives complained that the most problematic overriding issue with dually diagnosed people
was of a mental health nature and thus should be addressed in this arena. Individuals from both professions professed ignorance and lack of training in the
other's field of expertise.

The assembled representatives agreed that effective planning and cooperation
was needed to eliminate juggling dually diagnosed individuals from one program
to another. As deinstitutionalization efforts progressed, a number of dually diagnosed people had increasingly come to the attention of community legal authorities due to their severe acting-out behaviors. The question of agency responsibility for people considered anomalies to the community system could no longer be
pushed aside.

Evolution and Outcomes of the DD-MH Consortium Model

The service provider representatives successfully secured a state grant to explore ways to address their mutual problems. With the aid of a consultant and community input during an open forum, the group developed seven recommendations, presented and discussed below.

Meet monthly and to call themselves the Pueblo DD-MH Consortium. The Consortium has now been meeting monthly for over 15 years and has reviewed more than 150 cases.

Rotate the site of monthly meetings between participating agencies. Initially the meeting site was rotated between participating agencies to help ensure equal "ownership" and involvement. As the group experienced the many benefits of their collaborative efforts, this soon became unnecessary. The group decided to meet regularly in a central location at the Colorado Mental Health Institute (formerly Colorado State Hospital).

Broadly define DD-MH people to include any "functionally retarded" individual with borderline or below intellectual functioning who was creating significant problems in the community. The Consortium members agreed to a broad definition of people with a dual diagnosis, including individuals with developmental disabilities who were also offenders. This initial "target population" has continued to be a primary focus. The Consortium has also expanded its role to address concerns that the judges have identified regarding people with significant mental illness who do not have developmental disabilities but who also come before the courts as offenders. In response to these concerns the Consortium appointed a mental health subcommittee, which has developed Project Intercept. This project addresses the issues of people with acute mental illness who have broken the law and who are in need of appropriate disposition. Project Intercept provides these individuals with the opportunity to volunteer to be included in a database that indicates that they would like to be assisted by a case manager from mental health services if they get in trouble with the law. This does not provide individuals with a carte blanch to commit crimes without consequences. On the contrary, this process provides the mentally ill offender with timely and professional assistance to address the need for medication or other psychiatric intervention while under arrest and incarcerated. This intervention process also does not eliminate the possibility that the individual may face charges and may have to go to jail until further disposition is determined. As a result of the case management intervention, however, the offender with mental illness is able to receive proper professional assistance and, it is hoped, some degree of stabilization in the interim. Project Intercept provides the individual with mental illness the opportunity for a case review and the potential for treatment provider recommendations to the courts for intervention.

Have the Consortium serve as an advisory board to respond to presentations regarding individuals placed in settings where services were proving to be inadequate.

The Consortium has played a major role in serving as an advisory board for presentations regarding individuals who may have been inappropriately placed in settings where services were inadequate to meet their needs. Additionally, the Consortium expanded its role to include other presentations related to crisis situations (e.g., aggressive outbursts, runaway behavior, theft, sexual acting out) and many other types of behavioral and psychiatric issues. A number of these presentations involved individuals who were brought before the court and were provided with a "creative sentencing" process that helps ensure that individuals receive consequences for their behavior that are appropriate and meaningful for them. This process is discussed in greater detail in a later section.

Expand membership to include advocates and legal system representatives. Membership has evolved and expanded over the years. Although the intent of the Consortium initially was to bring together professionals and staff from agencies serving people with developmental disabilities and mental health needs, representatives from a third professional field, criminal justice, were soon included. Participants from the criminal justice system have included the assistant district attorney, sheriff's representatives, the chief of police and other officers, Probation and Parole representatives, and representatives from the Public Defender's Office. The assistant district attorney and the chief of police have been consistent representatives and have been invaluable in addressing criminal justice legal requirements and issues that offenders with developmental disabilities face while being processed through the criminal justice system.

Use the Consortium to educate others as successful solutions to mutual problems were found. Educating others has been an important goal of the Consortium. The inclusion of criminal justice representatives has also led to the opportunity for the Consortium to provide in-service training to police officers, sheriffs' deputies, assistant district attorneys, public defenders, and probation officers. To date, the Consortium has provided police training to more than 100 officers and has trained 136 sheriffs' deputies and approximately 40 assistant district attorneys. Additionally, Consortium members have met with public defenders' staffs and have offered assistance in working with people with developmental disabilities. Several probation officers who were assigned to work with individuals with special needs have also been trained. Material covered in the training sessions has included: (a) what is mental retardation? (b) differences between mental retardation and mental illness, (c) how an officer can determine if an individual has a developmental disability, (d) the rights of a person with a developmental disability as opposed to individuals without a developmental disability as they relate to the criminal justice system, (e) how a probation officer can help an individual with a developmental disability without demeaning the individual, (f) whether or not people with a developmental disability should experience consequences for their behavior, (g) how to avoid reinforcing repetitive problem behaviors that require law-enforcement intervention, and (h) whom to contact if an arrested individual is suspected of having a developmental disability. A final and very beneficial educational effort within the criminal justice system has come in the form of dinner meetings. The Consortium has hosted several dinners with local judges creating the opportunity to develop these relationships further and to discuss the progress the system has been making with offenders with a developmental disability in Pueblo. In addition to the specific training for law enforcement officials, the Consortium has sponsored three different workshops involving presenters from eastern Michigan, Pennsylvania, and Massachusetts. These workshops were attended by representatives from all the participating agencies involved in the Consortium. Topics included a retrospective workshop on the Consortium, a workshop featuring the Lancaster, Pennsylvania, program that deals with individuals with developmental disabilities who have become criminal offenders, people with developmental disabilities who are mistreated while incarcerated, and individuals with developmental disabilities who have received the death penalty.

Support the formation of a DD offender program. The initiation of a project for intensive specialized community-based services for offenders with a developmental disability began in 1989. Colorado Bluesky Enterprises (then the Pueblo County Board for Development Disabilities) was chosen to design and oversee the project. The DD-MH Consortium provided the impetus and the initial support within the criminal justice system for a one-bed pilot facility to appear viable. Components of the Resocialization Through Understanding, Limits, Training, and Support (RESULTS) Program (previously called the DD Offender Program) included residential and vocational services as well as specialized case management and psychological services. Further description of this program and its outcomes is provided later in this chapter.

Cooperative efforts among members of the Consortium have exceeded expectations. Members of the Consortium have helped individuals into temporary placements from one service agency to another as part of the plan to help an individual become stabilized. All representatives from their respective agencies have worked to ensure there is no "dumping" of individuals. By presenting an individual's case to the Consortium, proper plans have been developed, and the various agency representatives have taken it upon themselves to offer assistance, knowing the agency with primary responsibility will continue to assume final responsibility for the individual. This has avoided the turf battles that service agencies experienced prior to the establishment of the Consortium. Over the years, great trust and respect have been established among the Consortium members; this has improved the services and supports each of the agencies offer individuals with developmental disability and mental health needs.

In addition to trust, the Consortium members speak of a camaraderie achieved among the members. The impact of this camaraderie has extended to other areas beyond the dually diagnosed and the offender with developmental disabilities and may have contributed to the longevity of the Consortium. Individual members frequently call on one another for advice or assistance for other issues their agency might be faced with (e.g., staff training, consultation on programs, grant endorsements). Members also have been called upon to help make presentations at state and national conferences regarding the DD-MH Consortium model. Due to the statewide reputation of the Consortium, many members include their Consortium membership on grants, vitas, and applications. Consortium members also have been given certificates of recognition at the annual Recognition Picnic of Colorado Bluesky Enterprises Inc. (CBE), one of the 20 community-centered boards in the state. This event is attended by 300 to 400 guests each year, many being elected officials and influential businesspeople. This has created public support for members' efforts and recognition beyond the Consortium's meeting room.

Consortium members have also consulted with professionals having problems with people with developmental disabilities in other communities in Colorado. In addition to consultation regarding specific cases, several communities have shown an interest in establishing a consortium. To date two other communities have actively begun a consortium model, and three other communities started consortia that did not last. Reasons given by some of the agency representatives where the model failed was a lack of interest, inconsistency in meetings, and the lack of commitment by any single agency to take responsibility for pulling the other agencies together. In Pueblo, Colorado, Bluesky Enterprises Inc. has taken that responsibility to help ensure the continued existence of such an effective collaboration.

The RESULTS Program

Over its 13 years of operation the Resocialization Through Understanding, Limits, Training, and Support (RESULTS) Program has expanded to three, three-bed, staffed homes and one additional placement in another three-bed staffed home. Several successful "graduates" have moved to less structured and more independent settings. The collaborative team process among the various components of the program as well as the coordination between DD-MH service providers and the legal system has worked well. People who are typically served within this program meet eligibility requirements for developmental disability services and have a mental health diagnosis (Axis I, per *Diagnostic and Statistical Manual of Mental Disorders,* 4th ed. [American Psychiatric Association, 1994]). Two homes serve men and a third home was opened the end of 2000 for three women. The majority of people served have a fairly extensive history of involvement in the criminal justice system, often to the extent of having been incarcerated for a lengthy period of time and/or on several different occasions. The offenses of individuals served have included burglary, assault with a deadly weapon, sexual assault on a child, harassment through obscene phone calls, stalking, and child abuse resulting in death.

Program Services

Residential services for these individuals are provided in a highly structured and closely supervised setting in suburban neighborhoods in the community. Each home serves a maximum of three individuals with one male staff member on duty at all times as well as one female staff member on duty at all times in the home for women. Double coverage is provided in all facilities on weekends and evenings to allow more opportunity for outings and appointments. Each individual is provided with an individualized point-level program, described below, which is adjusted as needed by the team on an ongoing basis. Vocational services are provided in an integrated community setting and are also an important component of the RESULTS Program. Work crews typically include three to five individuals and one supervisor. Jobs include ground maintenance service, cleaning a veterinary business, parking structure cleanup, and other active work.

Vocational services include the provision of extensive structure and supervision as well as daily communication with residential staff and other team members as needed. In 2000 a RESULTS day program was developed for a few of the women and men served in the RESULTS residential program who have continued to have severe assaultive and run-away behavior when working on mobile crews in the community. This program primarily takes place on a seven-acre farm and involves work in the areas of gardening; yard work; sanding and other woodworking activities; painting; and caring for a variety of animals, including miniature horses, chickens, dogs, and pigs. The opportunity for more desirable chores and increased wages increases as individuals move up on their program level.

Case management services are also highly specialized and require a case manager with a good working knowledge of the criminal justice system and behavioral programming as well as an added time commitment as an integral member of the RESULTS Program team. The case manager is frequently involved in case presentations to the DD-MH Consortium and is generally the person who negotiates sentencing recommendations among the team, district attorney, and public defender.

Psychological services include coordination of the RESULTS team and responsibility for the development of an individualized behavioral point-level program for each individual served. Individual and group psychotherapy services are also provided or coordinated by the team psychologist. An Appropriate Social and Sexual Expression Therapy (ASSET) group is cofacilitated by the CBE psychologist and the CBE chief executive officer. This weekly group includes eight men who have a history of sexual offenses, many against children.

Initial and continued education for people working directly with individuals served within the RESULTS Program begins with an extensive 16-unit training orientation and an additional 16-unit training package. Training topics include applied learning theory, background in mental health, offender and sexual offender issues, and methods to deescalate and contain physical aggression. On-the-job training, periodic workshops, and involvement in the team process are an integral part of training as well. People working directly with individuals in the RESULTS Program are those who have demonstrated the ability to respond to individuals served with the full range of firm direction and sensitivity required by this challenging population. At the same time these staff members are also physically capable of dealing with individuals who may be physically assaultive.

Team Focus

A cohesive team approach with a focus on proactive planning and ongoing communication is a major hallmark of the RESULTS Program. Team members in each of the three residential facilities include four to six full-time staff members and their supervisor as well as the individual receiving services. Other team members include the individual's work supervisor, the individual's case manager, and a psychologist. In the case of those individuals receiving services who are on parole or probation, the parole or probation officer is also an important member of the team, communicating with the team once or twice a month.

Before a person enters the RESULTS Program, each team member typically meets with the person individually in his or her current setting to become acquainted, discuss the individuals goals, behavioral issues, potential reinforcers, and so forth. Additionally, the individual will also meet with the team several days prior to placement to provide additional input into the point-level program, to become somewhat familiar with the team meeting process, and to discuss further information regarding the overall plan for treatment. The very important concept that the individual and all team members are working together in close communication is conveyed to the individual verbally as well as in practice. This practice is stressed in an effort to maximize program consistency and to minimize the opportunity for manipulation on the part of the individual served.

When an individual moves into a RESULTS residential facility, he or she begins earning, losing, and spending points according to the parameters of their individualized point-level program. The point-level system involves a series of levels from 5 (lowest and least amount of privileges) to Level 1 (most independent). Each level, with the accompanying responsibilities, privileges, and criteria for movement to that level are specified in a detailed written program. Levels 5, 4, 3, and often 2 typically include a token economy that provides the opportunity for the individual to earn points to spend for privileges, chosen from a list of available options developed with input from the individual served and the team.

Points, as well as a level, may also be lost for specified behavior problems. Level 1 involves a check sheet of responsibilities and privileges that the staff, as well as the individual, maintains.

For a minimum of the first 2 days after placement, an individual will typically remain in the residential facility on program Level 5, to begin the transition from jail or prison into a slightly less physically structured yet more behaviorally demanding setting. During this time the individual and staff have the opportunity to become better acquainted, to experience the individual's response to the point-level program, and to recommend necessary program adjustments to the team as needed.

After a minimum of 2 days on Level 5 with no point loss, the individual is eligible to move to Level 4. This level generally includes the opportunity to go to work as well as to participate in outings in the community with close one-to-one supervision. In some cases residential staff may accompany the individual to work for several days or more depending on the degree of vocational supervision available and the severity of the individual's challenging behavior.

Individuals may move from Level 4 up through each level by successfully maintaining their behavior without point loss for approximately 1 to 2 months, depending on the level. Team consensus for level advancement is also required. Each higher level involves increased responsibilities and privileges with an eventual goal of fading staff supervision as the individual demonstrates a greater degree of trustworthiness and self-control.

Team members meet regarding each individual on a bimonthly basis for approximately 45 minutes to discuss all aspects of each person's previous 2 weeks. Summary reports are presented by residential and vocational staff; these include data related to the point-level program with more detailed comments if points have been lost during the week. The individual's concerns and questions for the team, staff impressions of overall progress, family contacts, outings with staff, and so forth, are also discussed. Individuals participate in team meetings and are assisted by staff in organizing their questions or concerns throughout the week.

In any situation where a team member questions the possibility of manipulation by the client, the team member is encouraged to bring the issue up for discussion at the team meeting, rather than immediately responding to the issue. This process continues to provide the individual with the clear message that staff members are working together with the individual as a team and that all major decisions are made by the entire team. Within the residential facility, staff members further enhance communication through a daily log of significant events. They also participate in change of shift meetings that provide the opportunity to elaborate on or further clarify these notes.

Outcomes

To date, the CBE RESULTS Program has served 22 individuals residentially and vocationally and four additional people in the Appropriate Social and Sexual Expression Therapy (ASSET) group. Three individuals were served only briefly due to elopement and a desire to return to former placements (e.g., home community, state hospital, and prison to complete a shorter sentence) and another was readmitted to the Pueblo Regional Center after a series of assaults on staff and housemates. One of the first individuals served by the RESULTS Program moved into his own apartment in May 1991, largely due to a "glitch" in the system that afforded him an early release from parole. This individual experienced intermittent problems, however, because he ultimately chose to terminate all support services in December 1993 and was incarcerated again in the spring of 2000.

Another individual was able to live alone and work in the community with no problems from May 1993 until March 2000, when a reoffense resulted in his return to the RESULTS Program and 24-hour supervision. Four other individuals successfully moved into personal care alternative (PCA) host homes, one in September 1994, one in June 1996 and two in December 1998. These individuals are living with families (without children) or companions and continue to meet with their support team on a monthly basis. Two other individuals completed successful transitions into a PCA home with families in their home communities. Additionally, two individuals have successfully moved into less structured, staffed PCAs, one in March 1997, and one in April 1999.

The 10 individuals currently being served in the RESULTS Program have each made significant gains. Although progress in some cases is slow, the intensive program has resulted in progress that is notable especially in light of the extensive problematic history of these individuals.

A number of successful outcomes have been noted among members of the ASSET group as well. Outcomes include three "graduates" of the group who live independently with drop-in supports and who have had no incidents of relapse, as well as three individuals from this group who have moved into less restrictive residential settings. In addition to the "target" outcomes that include very rare and relatively minor reoffenses, increased honesty, and ability to take responsibility for behavior, some surprises have also occurred. Several group members have increased their reading skills dramatically as a result of homework assignments that involve writing down progress toward a weekly goal. The ability to focus and to shift attention away from visual stimuli (e.g., a child) or "stinking thinking" has also been remarkable in some group members. Social skills have increased considerably as have expressions of true concern and encouragement among group members.

Another key objective of the RESULTS Program has been to provide each individual with a lengthy period of success in this structured environment and a very gradual transition into a less structured and carefully selected home. At times this can be difficult to adhere to, given the great need for these types of services by other individuals. Strong administrative support, which does not succumb to the pressure to dilute the long-term effectiveness of this program for an individual through premature movement, has also been a critical factor in the success of this program. This support is empowering to RESULTS team members as they are able to experience the rewards of making a significant difference in the lives of each individual served.

In dealing with this highly challenging population, it is important to revisit our definition of *success* to enhance the morale of individuals served as well as preserving that of service providers. Increased time without an offense or decreased severity of an offense, as well as positive changes in interpersonal and work skills, must be applauded. Proactive efforts to educate key players in the criminal justice system, including judges and district attorneys, as well as parole, probation, and detention officers, has been another key factor in the success of the RESULTS Program. Currently a primary effort is being made to consequate early, relatively minor offenses of individuals with developmental disabilities in a manner intended to be meaningful in terms of preventing future occurrences of unlawful behavior. The tremendous collaborative efforts of the Pueblo DD-MH Consortium members in this project cannot be overstated.

New Challenges and Initiatives

Over the 15 years of the Pueblo Consortium's existence, new challenges have come to the attention of the group. As the cohesiveness and mutual trust of the group developed, the spirit of proactive planning and creative program implementation has flourished.

A major accomplishment of the Consortium has been the development of a process to address the disposition of the offender with developmental disabilities while in the criminal justice system. This process provides criminal justice officials with a contact person, the individual's case manager, who is responsible for helping the officials determine how to provide an appropriate and effective plan for disposition of the individual offender. Case managers, who work with the developmental disabilities service agency, are available on a 24-hour, on-call basis 365 days of the year that has helped strengthen the communication and cooperative relationship between the criminal justice system and developmental disabilities services. Case managers are able to provide a timely response to law enforcement personnel and, after consultation with the individual's team and, in many instances, the Consortium, are able to recommend a well-developed plan for sentencing to the judge. The implementation of "creative sentencing" has been a key part of the process that ensures that the judges have recommendations for alternative dispositions that have a consequence specific to each individual. This process has been invaluable in ensuring that individuals served in the RESULTS Program receive consequences for their behavior that are appropriate and meaningful for each individual.

The issue of competency to stand trial has also been addressed by the Pueblo Consortium. Prior to the establishment of the Consortium, many individuals with developmental disabilities had been inappropriately sent to the forensic unit at the Colorado Mental Health Institute — Pueblo (CMHI--P) as a consequence for their offenses. The forensic unit houses hard-core offenders with a mental illness. Offenders with developmental disabilities sometime suffered abuse from mainstream inmates and such incidents were rarely reported to authorities, because of a code of silence and intolerance to "snitches." It had been obvious to forensic mental health professionals that the needs of the more typical inmates were not compatible with the needs of the offender with developmental disabilities. Therefore the job of protecting these individuals from being harmed or used by other inmates was an overwhelming burden the mental health workers assumed reluctantly. Consortium members discovered that labeling certain individuals with developmental disabilities as Incompetent to Proceed (ITP) was, in many cases, giving that individual a life sentence on the forensic unit, because some offenders with a developmental disability could not pass the competency test. By avoiding the issue of competency in the courts, and with creative sentencing, the individual could be provided with meaningful consequences and not lose his or her freedom (personal rights) on a long-term basis. Additionally, the forensic unit at the CMHI--P was relieved of the frustration and responsibility of trying to deal with the many offenders with developmental disabilities previously brought to that institution.

The Consortium has also recently developed Project ASSIST (Assault, Safety, and Social Intervention Systems Training). This project is similar to Project Intercept, described earlier, which addresses the issues of people with acute mental illness who have broken the law and are in need of assistance from a mental health case manager. Project ASSIST provides a voluntary, centralized identification and tracking system for individuals with developmental disabilities who are classified as offenders or those who may otherwise come to the attention of law enforcement officers or emergency psychiatric or medical personnel due to behavior that is a danger to self or others. Individuals with medical conditions, such as seizures or uncontrolled diabetes, or problems with drug or alcohol abuse may also be included in the tracking system. A contact number is made available to police and sheriff dispatch personnel for immediately accessing critical information and understanding about individuals who may be "picked up" on the street by law enforcement personnel or who may be reported by program staff in need of police or sheriff assistance. Details of this process are shared with the criminal justice system through training sessions and the involvement of law enforcement personnel in Consortium meetings.

The innovative planning efforts of the Pueblo Consortium continue to expand to meet new challenges as they arise. In a time of increasing attention to paper and red tape, the creative, solution-focused spirit of the group serves as a breath of fresh air for everyone involved.

Case Study

Five case studies as well as much of the information highlighted in this chapter are discussed in greater detail in a manual titled *The Pueblo DD-MH Consortium Story: Documentation of a Community Voluntary Collaborative Effort, A Training Manual* written by Larry Velasco, with contributions by Lamar Trant and Peter Holmes (Velasco, 1993). A case summary and update are provided here to illustrate typical responses to the Consortium's program and treatment.

Carl (fictitious name) had a triple concern regarding the challenges he was facing. He had diagnoses of pedophilia, same-sex, nonexclusive type, and fragile X syndrome, and he was also a person diagnosed as having a developmental disability. Carl had received services and supports since he was a child, receiving his education in a segregated school for developmentally disabled children in a small rural community in Colorado. He was placed in a foster care home at a very early age. He remained in foster care until he was 16 years old, when he was allowed to move back home with his mother, step-dad and half sister. That same year his family moved to a metropolitan city and, shortly thereafter, he was charged with sexual assault on a male child. Carl avoided criminal charges but had civil charges filed against him, resulting in him being imposed into an institution for people with developmental disabilities. He remained in the institution for 6 years and was subsequently moved to a personal care alternative host home program in Pueblo. Carl was moved a number of times by the agency providing him services, thus experiencing a very unstable living situation for several more years. He was also reported to have made sexual advances toward male children in some of these settings.

In 1989 the police were called because a parent complained that Carl had offered two young boys money to take their clothes off and lie on each other. No charges were filed in this case. In February 1990 Carl was left alone with a 7-year-old grandson of his PCA provider and Carl reportedly offered the boy money for oral sex. Unfortunately, the incident was not reported for 3 days. When Carl was confronted by the administrators of the service agency, he ran away. He ran away again after he was returned to the provider and refused to cooperate with the program. Because no one knew what to do with Carl, he was admitted to the psychiatric ward of a local hospital in Pueblo.

Carl also had a history of problems with explosive behavior, flying into a rage with staff over the most minute incidents. He was tested and diagnosed with fragile X syndrome by the Fragile X Syndrome Project at Sewel Rehabilitation Center in Denver. The Fragile X Project personnel informed the staff that Carl had to have a calm environment and needed to be trained in calming himself down when he started to become anxious. The Fragile X Project report also requested that Carl receive 24-hour supervision to help him deal with his fragile X challenges in a more effective manner. The staff was also alerted that psychotropic medications tend to have a reverse effect on individuals with fragile X, causing them to be more irritable and out of control. Additional program recommendations were made for eliciting more favorable behavioral responses from Carl and avoiding the power plays and unnecessary stressors that come with power plays. Unfortunately, the agency providing Carl with services was having a number of personnel problems, resulting in high staff turnover which added to Carl's problems. Apparently the recommendations made by the Fragile X Project were not implemented, resulting in an escalation of Carl's sexual and assaultive problems to the point where he became completely uncontrollable. In one instance Carl locked the staff out of the apartment, made loud, threatening phone calls, and "trashed" the apartment. In another instance he threw chairs and ashtrays at the staff. Finally, Carl began making obscene phone calls; police were called in, and Carl yelled and cursed at them and had to be physically restrained but, again, was not arrested.

In 1993 Carl was presented to the DD-MH Consortium at the request of the Human Rights Committee, which exhorted the staff to intervene in a more effective manner before Carl or others were severely hurt. Carl was placed in the Pueblo Regional Center state-operated residential facility for 10 days and an Imposition of Legal Disability was instituted by the case management agency at the recommendation of the Consortium. Carl was ultimately placed in the RESULTS Program with two other individuals receiving services. This program provided structure and 24-hour supervision and helped Carl enroll in the Appropriate Social and Sexual Expression Therapy (ASSET) group for sex offenders as well as individual therapy once a week. Carl also was restricted from contact with children at all times. Additionally, Carl was provided with a calm, structured environment in which decisions were made by the entire RESULTS Program team. The biweekly team meetings and decision-making eliminated disjointed decisions and any opportunity for manipulation on Carl's part. Carl was involved in a contractual relationship with the team through his point-level program, thereby making it clear to him what was expected of him at all times. This program also provided Carl with an opportunity to participate in identifying goals and reinforcers that he would work to achieve. He learned that he could lose reinforcers and could have his goals delayed as a consequence of his behavior.

Carl was enrolled in the RESULTS Program in 1993, and by 1996 he had worked so hard and improved to such an extent that he was allowed to interview and select a PCA host home provider whom he lived with for 3 years. Carl and his team selected a male provider who was a bachelor at the time. This was somewhat of a difficult transition for Carl in that he had to learn a whole new lifestyle with this particular person. The transition process was carried out in a systematic manner, however, with numerous visits in Carl's home as well as his potential provider's home. Additionally, his team continued to meet with Carl on a monthly, or more frequent as-needed basis, to review issues, needed program changes, and to train and support the new provider. Carl became involved in his provider's softball games, learning about outfielding, and hitting the ball and became a favorite assistant to the team. Carl was also involved with the provider's parents' family activities where he had the opportunity to eat ethnic Mexican food — and loved it. He was also included in anniversary and holiday celebrations and was a member of the wedding party when his provider got married in 1998. This transition was also initially challenging for Carl but was dealt with openly, as Carl became better at expressing his feelings.

As mentioned previously, Carl was involved in the Appropriate Social and Sexual Expression Therapy group with seven other peers. In the beginning Carl would come to group therapy with a variety of somatic complaints. He would have a headache, eye ache, arm ache, leg ache, and laryngitis and would complain of these aches much of the time during group therapy. His therapists and other group members quickly learned to ignore these complaints and reinforce discussions of his activities and feelings. Carl's personality blossomed, and he became someone who was listened to as a result of his honest feedback and, at times, humorous quips and responses. After a year Carl no longer needed to attempt to gain attention with his somatic complaints, and he became the "friend" everyone in group liked to have.

In January 1999 Carl and his team received disappointing news. Carl's provider's wife was pregnant, and Carl had to face the ordeal of having his life disrupted once again due to circumstances beyond his control. Although he became appropriately emotional at the prospect of losing his family of 3 years, he realized he could not remain in a home with an infant. He expressed himself well in group and in individual therapy and was able to cooperate with the process of finding another provider whom he and his team selected. As fortune would have it, Carl selected a provider who had another consumer living in the home who was also involved in the ASSET group with Carl and with whom Carl got along well. Carl was elated that he found an ideal housemate and family to move in with. He stated in group with a big smile, "I'm so happy."

During the entire time Carl has been in therapy and in the RESULTS Program (8 years), he has had zero incidents of sexual perpetration. He is learning to deal with his "stinking thinking" and has found other outlets for his energy and emotional expression. Over the past 9 years, Carl has had a few incidents in which he lost his temper and refused to talk with his host home provider or his job training supervisor; however, his reactions were more appropriate and did not escalate to the point of a need for police intervention. Carl loses privileges when he violates his behavior contract and clearly understands the consequences of his behavior. The frequency of these losses has been low, because Carl has learned self-control techniques, which he has applied himself. One of Carl's practices to get himself under control has been listening to a relaxation tape, provided by his group therapist. His therapist also provided him with opera tapes, which he loves. Although Carl has progressed a great deal during these past 9 years, his therapists and team realize Carl will always need some form of supervision. He himself has stated that he never wants to live on his own. His team's goal is to emancipate Carl to the extent that he is able to experience life to the fullest without reverting to the problematic behavior that plagued his early life. To this date Carl has demonstrated much growth and maturity and is a great model and inspiration to his peers.

References

American Psychiatric Association. (1994). *Diagnostic and statistical manual of mental disorders* (4th ed.). Washington, DC: Author.

Colorado Department of Human Services. (1999, March 4). *Office of Health and Rehabilitation/Direct Services, Developmental Disabilities Program, FY 1999–2000 Figure Setting* (JBC Working Document), p. 12.

Fidura, J. G., Lindsey, E. R., & Walker, G. R. (1987). A special behavior unit for treatment of behavior problems of persons who are mentally retarded. *Mental Retardation, 25,* 107–111.

Lord, J., & Pedlar, A. (1991). Life in the community: Four years after the closure of an institution. *Mental Retardation, 29,* 213–221.

Menolascino, F. J., Gilson, S. F., & Levitas, A. S. (1986). Issues in the treatment of mentally retarded patients in the community mental health system. *Community Mental Health Journal, 22,* 314–327.

Szymanski, L. S. (1987). Prevention of psychosocial dysfunction in persons with mental retardation. *Mental Retardation, 25,* 215–218.

Velasco, L. A. (1993). *The Pueblo DD-MH Consortium Story: Documentation of a Community Voluntary Collaborative Effort, A Training Manual.* Pueblo, CO: Pueblo DD-MH Consortium.

CHAPTER 9

Training and Technical Assistance Strategies to Prevent and Respond to Behavior-Related Crises

Daniel J. Baker
Karen Craven
Oregon Rehabilitation Association
Salem, Oregon

Richard W. Albin
University of Oregon
Eugene, Oregon

Norman A. Wieseler
Eastern Minnesota Community Support Services
Faribault, Minnesota

The request is familiar to anyone who has provided technical assistance or consultation related to behavior crisis intervention. *Teach us how to hold him or her down!* When support providers are (or see themselves as being) at physical risk, it is not surprising that the first thing they want to know is how to restrain someone. However, behavior specialists and crisis intervention training packages should present physical intervention and restraint as a last resort. The continued need for restraint is one indicator that behavior support plans and processes are not working adequately. Training for support providers in topics related to behavior crises must emphasize proactive supports and prevention. Reactive strategies may be necessary, but are not the primary components of a comprehensive approach to behavior crisis prevention and intervention.

A behavioral crisis frequently provides the impetus for a support agency, family, or other provider to seek training or technical assistance. Unfortunately, this casts such efforts, particularly the provision of technical assistance, in a reactive mode. This chapter provides an overview of a comprehensive approach to crisis prevention and intervention with an emphasis on positive behavior support strategies and proactive systems for staff training and staff support. This chapter is organized around the following topics: (a) definitions of crisis, (b) levels of crisis response, (c) types of support for people in crisis, (d) models of technical assistance, (e) training for care providers, (f) identification of people at risk, (g) reactive assistance, and (h) evaluation.

Definition of Crisis

In considering crisis supports, it is important to first define what constitutes a crisis. The authors define a crisis as a situation in which a person is engaging in behaviors that: (a) present a threat to the health and safety of the individual or others, or (b) may result in the person losing his or her home, job, access to activities, and community involvement. Behavioral crises are among the greatest challenges faced by agencies or care providers for individuals with developmental disabilities. Whereas this book is focused primarily upon behavioral crises, the authors of this chapter point out the commonalities between behavioral and other types of crisis in support needs, training strategies, and technical assistance approaches. Types of crises commonly encountered by care providers include (a) behavioral, (b) psychiatric, (c) medical, and (d) sexual aggression.

Levels of Crisis Response

Some are more urgent than others. Some can be detected as they gradually emerge, allowing support providers to plan their response. Others may not be detected in early stages or may escalate very quickly, reducing the planned preparedness. The immediacy of response will depend on the type of difficulty and range in three levels.

Level 1: An immediate response is necessary. Support may need to be added or placement changed in less that 24 hours.

Level 2: Intense assistance is necessary between one day and one month from the time of referral.

Level 3: Moderate assistance is necessary, but the crisis is not likely to result in short-term displacement. The solutions are likely to be long term in both nature and effect.

Each of these three levels of response calls for different training and technical assistance needs. It is important to know the level of response necessary in planning interventions. Ideally, all support agencies and providers would have the capacity to respond effectively to any level of crisis. In reality, agencies, families, and other support providers often do not have the capacity to respond adequately using existing "internal" (i.e., available within an agency or local system) resources. Clinicians or consultants often are called in to help ameliorate the difficulties being encountered as a result of the behavior crisis. The many different definitions of consultant (e.g., Kratochwill & Bergen, 1990) do agree that a consultant is an expert in the topic area (e.g., behavior support or mental illness) who assists care providers in solving problems related to supporting the individual. The consultant is not a current service or care provider or a regular member of the support team for a person with disabilities. Even in agencies that do employ their own behavior specialist and rely on this person as a resource to deal with crises, it is likely that this specialist-consultant is (at least nominally) from "outside" the regular support team. The need to go outside regular support teams for assistance, and the nature of the consultant relationship with the regular support team, have implications for the provision of training and technical assistance to prevent and respond to crises.

Services a Consultant Can Provide

Whether from inside or outside a support agency, a consultant or behavior specialist is likely to provide services in the form of training or technical assistance. On some occasions a consultant may also be expected to provide hands-on support or direct intervention. A major goal of training or technical assistance is to increase the capacity of an agency or support provider to accomplish desired outcomes, such as being able to: (a) safely and effectively respond to behavioral crisis and (b) prevent and avoid the occurrence of behavioral crisis. Although related and sometimes combined, the authors find it useful to distinguish between training and technical assistance.

In training situations, the consultant will assist and enhance capacity by raising the knowledge and skill level of care providers, typically by engaging in activities designed to result in the "audience" learning new information and skills. Common examples include workshops, lectures, or other forms of teaching, but may also include coaching or mentoring. Training also may involve the introduction of new forms or materials that trainees can use.

In technical assistance situations, the consultant provides more direct assistance and produces products designed for intended use in different interventions and support strategies, resulting in specific recommendations for improving behavior support for an individual. The consultant takes direct responsibility for certain, prespecified outcomes, such as conducting a functional assessment or writing a behavior support plan. Capacity is increased immediately by the presence of a highly skilled consultant. However, to enhance capacity after the consultant's responsibilities are ended, it is important that some training of "regular" support team members occurs; that is, technical assistance should include training.

Although it is common to seek the services of a consultant or specialist to respond to a current crisis, we strongly recommend using training and/or technical assistance in a manner that balances proactive and reactive intervention in addressing crises. A common mistake in providing behavioral support is waiting until a situation turns into a major behavioral crisis before seeking help (i.e., staff training or technical assistance). We use the word proactive to refer to things done before a problem behavior emerges or escalates in intensity to crisis level. An example of a proactive intervention is to schedule easy tasks among difficult tasks if doing too many difficult tasks in a row causes problem behaviors (Horner, Day, Sprague, O'Brien, & Heathfield, 1991; Mace et al., 1988). We use the word reactive to refer to things done once the problem behavior occurs. An example of a reactive intervention is to ask a person to go to a quieter place when he or she "acts out." It is a well-established axiom that the best crisis response is to prevent crises from occurring in the first place.

Steps in Training and Technical Assistance

A consultant might provide a number of services to assist an agency or support provider. The first step in technical assistance is defining the problem. People involved in a crisis often are not able to accurately define the crisis. They may know that a severe problem exists, but may have difficulties describing it. This often happens when care providers are emotionally involved or distracted by other things and, as a result, lose objectivity and the ability to observe events clearly. An external person, such as a consultant, can lend objectivity in defining the situation. The following example illustrates this situation.

An individual was reported to bite himself at seemingly unpredictable times. A consultant went to observe him at his worksite. A wireless phone was on the table next to him. The phone rang, and the individual immediately began to bite himself. He had a very frightened look on his face. The staff person did not notice this, though, because he was on the phone. After the incident was over, the staff person expressed puzzlement as to why the individual bit himself. The staff person missed the link between the self-injury and the phone call.

A second type of service a consultant might provide is to help regular support team members identify why the problem exists. A key element of current positive behavioral support approaches is an emphasis on designing and implementing support strategies that are based on and logically linked to hypotheses regarding why and when problem behaviors occur and what maintains them (Horner, 1999a; Horner, Albin, Sprague, & Todd, 1999b). A functional assessment is the most common way to identify reasons for problem behaviors. A functional assessment identifies the causal factors and maintaining variables associated with a problem behavior (Mace, 1994; chap. 10, this volume). Whereas functional assessment represents a formal process for identifying why a problem occurs, other less formal types of evaluation may be performed in crisis situations when time is of the essence (Rudolph, Lakin, Oslund, & Larson, 1998; Sprague, Flannery, O'Neill, & Baker, 1996). More formal, controlled types of functional assessment, such as structured, direct observation or functional analyses, can be performed if causes for problem behavior are difficult to discern (Horner, 1994; Repp, 1999; Shores, Wehby, & Jack, 1999).

Third, a consultant can help develop a behavior support plan, especially a comprehensive behavior support plan. This topic will be developed further in following sections of this chapter, but, in short, a behavior support plan represents steps in preventing and responding to problems or crises and improving behavior support strategies. A behavior support plan should have both proactive and reactive elements (O'Neill et al., 1997).

Fourth, a consultant can train and support people who implement the plan, whether family members, support staff, or other types of care providers. Training for care providers and raising skill levels are among the most crucial of elements in supporting, resolving, and preventing crises (Baker, 1998; Foxx, 1996; Sprague et al., 1996). However, this is often beyond the scope of consultation (Foxx, 1996).

Fifth, a consultant with expertise in behavioral interventions and support can train, counsel, and support the person presenting the problem behavior. In other words, the consultant can support the individual directly. This can be useful in its direct effects on the person presenting the crisis and may indirectly benefit other care providers through modeling appropriate interactions and relationships. This may be time-intensive and is often prohibitively expensive.

Sixth, and finally, an external consultant can help identify relevant support services, especially if the consultant is familiar with resources in the community. Examples of resources include drug and alcohol counselors, therapists, psychiatric support services, and respite opportunities for care providers. Such assistance is typically very welcome.

Appropriate Roles and Balances

In any consulting activity, an appropriate balance of activities must be obtained, and roles must be identified before support services begin. Consultants may be asked to do far more than is appropriate to the situation or engage in activities beyond the scope of consultation. The following example presents one such situation.

A consultant was working with a foster home that employed a shift staff person. In the process of observation, the consultant noted the staff person exhibiting some patterns of interaction that led to escalations in problem behaviors.

When the consultant shared this with the foster family, they asked the consultant to fire the shift staff person for them.

Similarly, the consultant may be asked to do too little or may not be given sufficient hours to complete the requested tasks. For example, the consultant may be asked to teach staff people how to restrain a person without also giving or teaching them positive interventions. Another inappropriate use of consultants is to have consultants write a behavior support plan simply to satisfy statutory requirements.

To avoid these difficult and compromising situations, the following recommendations are made: (a) establish a statement of work prior to beginning consultation, (b) establish fees and time limits, (c) establish a point of contact with the family or agency, (d) clearly delineate responsibilities, and (e) have the statement of work agreed to and signed by all parties. If the scope of work is not completely known prior to beginning the consultation, we recommend establishing an initial statement of work to explore the problem, and then setting a subsequent meeting to review proposed activities and finalize a statement of work.

Finally, in establishing roles and responsibilities, it is important that the consultant work collaboratively with existing support team members to address issues and problem solve. A common mistake in bringing in a consultant to address a behavioral crisis or behavioral support issues is to hand the "problem" to the consultant and say simply, "Fix this." Consultants may have high levels of technical knowledge and skills, but they should not be expected to singlehandedly identify and deliver the solution to a problematic situation. Nor would it be desirable for a consultant to assume the role of sole "fixer" of an agency's or support team's behavioral support problems (e.g., behavioral crisis). Regular support team members have essential information about the person in crisis (or at risk for crisis) and the person's situation and living conditions. Regular team members also have ongoing roles and responsibilities related to providing effective support, including the ability to prevent and respond to a behavioral crisis. Effective and sustainable plans and procedures to prevent and respond to a crisis are best developed and implemented in the context of a collaborative team process that uses the knowledge and strengths of regular team members and consultants.

Essential Components of Technical Assistance

Although there are various models that can be used in training and technical assistance (Kratochwill & Bergen, 1990), a few key features are seen across most successful consulting models. These are presented in Table 9.1. First, there should be a collegial, well-defined relationship between the consultant-technical assistance provider and the consumers of the consultation, with a written consultation agreement approved by all stakeholders. This agreement should include measures for ongoing support and organizational development, and should address the customers' desired outcomes and identify the indicators used to determine if goals are met. Common problems to consider in advance are: (a) whether an excessive emphasis is placed on the person with disabilities as the primary focus of problems, (b) whether training is possible, (c) whether resources are available, and (d) whether care providers are willing to make efforts, such as collecting data or changing interaction strategies. An ongoing, positive relationship between the consultant and the care providers will allow for better follow-up and reduce the chance of future relapses of problem behavior. An ongoing relationship also increases the consultant's opportunities to develop and foster a proactive orientation to support among the care providers. Assessments should always drive intervention efforts, and development of plans should be included in consultation efforts. Proactive plans for follow-up and evaluation are key elements of successful technical assistance.

Six-Step Model for Technical Assistance

We propose a six-step model for technical assistance in behavior support: (a) assessment procedures, (b) plan development, (c) plan implementation, (d) plan evaluation, (e) plan maintenance, and (f) organizational development.

Comprehensive Assessment

Comprehensive assessment involves two types of assessment activities. The first type involves environmental assessments and systems analyses designed to: (a) collect information on the settings in which a person lives and works (e.g., what fea-

---

TABLE 9.1
Essential Components of Technical Assistance

- Collaborative relationships
- Well-defined roles
- Ongoing relationship
- Comprehensive assessment
- Assessment drives intervention
- Plan development
- Follow-up
- Evaluation

tures work well, what features are problematic), (b) identify barriers to improving services and behavioral support, and (c) assess the local system to identify internal leadership, expertise, and needs for organizational development. In addition, information should be collected on the person with disabilities through a review of records and conversations with knowledgeable informants (including the person with disabilities, if appropriate) to identify both personal history information and plans, goals, or visions for the future (e.g., person-centered or future plans). Environmental and systems assessment information may be used to drive changes in physical, social, or programmatic features of living settings that may promote or contribute to occurrence of problem behaviors and behavioral crises.

The second type of assessment activity is conducting a functional behavioral assessment (FA) (see chap. 10, this volume). The outcomes of a functional behavioral assessment should include hypotheses regarding predictors and triggers of problem behaviors, setting events that increase the likelihood of problem behaviors, and the consequences or functions that maintain problem behaviors (Horner et al., 1999b; O'Neill et al., 1997).

The assessment phase should conclude by presenting the functional assessment hypothesis statements to the stakeholders and consumers, so that the whole support team may reach a consensus on where, when, and why problem behaviors occur (O'Neill et al., 1997; Sprague et al., 1996). Conducting and presenting the FA provides opportunities for training the team on topics regarding positive behavior support.

Plan Development

The second phase is plan development, which should occur in collaboration with the people who will be implementing the plan. The plan development phase should consider both needs and capacity of the site, and logistical ability to implement interventions (Baker, Dean, & Sprague, 1997; Kratochwill & Bergen, 1990; Sprague et al., 1996). Leverage point logic is recommended: Where can care providers get the most impact for their efforts? Where will efforts result in widespread effect? A problem-solving approach should be used as well, with an eye toward long-range planning (Kratochwill & Bergen).

Plan Implementation

Once the plan is developed, implementation is the next logical step. Key features involve developing a plan for implementation, reviewing the amount of support needed for implementation, assessing current capacity, providing training and support to meet needs and overcome deficits, and working collaboratively with the support team to assure that implementation works for them and that the support plans and processes are sustainable (Foxx, 1996; Lucyshyn & Albin, 1993; Sprague et al., 1996). To the maximum extent possible, the technical assistance provider should provide hands-on support for initial implementation and should be available to help trouble-shoot data collection mechanisms (Krachtowill & Bergen, 1990; Hughes & DeForest, 1993).

Plan Evaluation

Plan evaluation is another responsibility of the technical assistance provider during initial phases. Plan evaluation should go beyond simple counting of problem behavior frequencies and should address lifestyle change (described later in this chapter), implementation process, consultation process, and continuous quality improvement (J. M. Albin, 1992; Baker, Dean, & Sprague, 1997; Deming, 1986).

Plan Maintenance

Plan maintenance involves redefining roles and responsibilities between the consultant and stakeholders. Plans for maintaining staff performance and training new staff should be considered as well. Continuing evaluation efforts and procedures for plan revisions are critically important. This may involve specifying a process for shifting responsibilities for plan evaluation and modification to the agency or support provider. Consultant involvement should be faded in a planned and efficient manner; considerations for fading consultant involvement include the effectiveness of the behavior support procedures and variables related to the capacity of the agency or support providers (Sprague et al., 1996). Also plans must be made for potential recurrence of problem behavior. It is important to anticipate and plan for future crises. Flexibility and variation in behavior support efforts may improve maintenance in interventions long term (Foxx, 1996).

Organizational Development

Organizational development involves training and leaving educational information for agency personnel, staff, or family members. Strategically leaving information or documents in a person's files is another recommended strategy. These types of efforts can serve to build organizational memory and increase the general capacity of the care providers to respond to the next behavioral challenge, as well as avoid future challenges.

Nondirective Consultations

Another consideration in the design of consultation is a "nondirective consultation model" (Baker, 1998; Hughes & DeForest, 1993; Rule, Fodor-Davis, Morgan, Salzberg, & Chen, 1990). In this model, rather than providing answers and directly generating materials and plans, the technical assistance provider presents general information and guides local people through the process of decision making and intervention design. Additional training is given as dictated by the situation and the type of problems being presented. This approach has been demonstrated to be effective in school settings (Hughes & DeForest, 1993; Rule, Fodor-Davis, Morgan, Salzberg, & Chen, 1990), residential, and vocational support settings (Baker, 1998).

Training for Care Providers

Throughout this chapter, training has been discussed as a role of the technical assistance provider. The following section briefly presents best practices in training. Efforts to train staff often are presented as a remedy for poor staff performance (Reid, Parsons, & Green, 1989; Snell, 1990). Staff training interventions are performed for the purpose of teaching staff how or why to perform certain activities. Training interventions commonly feature instructional methods such as lectures, workshops, verbal and written instructions, staff assignments, and media-based presentation of information (J. M. Albin, Buckley, & Lynch, 1992). Supervised modeling, coaching, and role-playing interventions also have been used (Acosta-Amad & Brethower, 1992; Arco, 1991). Training often includes multiple components (e.g., Burch, Reiss, & Bailey, 1987). Nearly all service providers engage in training activities for staff, and most states require certain levels of in-service and preservice training (Larson, Hewitt, & Lakin, 1994). Ongoing, well-documented high levels of turnover in residential support settings create situations in which preservice training occurs on a very frequent, if not constant, basis (Braddock & Mitchell, 1992), rendering training new staff a nearly continual task. Clearly, staff training is a significant task and expense for providers.

When presenting new information, it is important to consider adult learning styles. In planning and presenting, trainers are encouraged to pay attention to the adult learning principles as presented in Table 9.2. Staff will learn more easily and retain more information if adult learning principles are considered (Wlodkowski, 1985).

Learners need to know how this new information or skill will make their lives better (Jensen, 1995). It is important to answer the question "Why do I need to know this?" and explain up front how the training will help them solve a problem or do their job better. The best training is "just in time," as knowledge is best retained when it is put to use immediately. The longer the delay between learning and use, the less effective the training will be, a theme common to all learners (Arco & Birnbrauer, 1990; Delameter, Connors, & Wells, 1994; Engelmann & Carnine, 1991; Jensen, 1995).

It is also important to build on existing knowledge and meaningfully relate the new information to the learners' previous experiences. For example, new staff people may have never considered the importance of providing choices to people with disabilities. But they can certainly relate to their own experiences of having

---

TABLE 9.2
Adult Learning Principles

Adults learn best when:

1. They are physically and mentally ready to focus on the information.

2. They see the learning as having personal value, meeting their goals.

3. The new material relates to past experiences.

4. They can see how the information can be applied in their lives and solve their problems.

5. Information is presented in a variety of learning modalities (e.g., auditory, visual, and kinesthetic).

6. They are actively involved in the process (e.g., physically, mentally, and emotionally).

7. They get helpful feedback to reinforce progress and correct poor performance.

8. They feel comfortable taking risks and experimenting with new knowledge and skills.

---

or not having control in their jobs or homes.

Trainers should train within or simulate the work environment whenever possible. Staff will be able to perform best on the job when the training conditions closely match the environment in which they will be working. For example, if staff typically needs to tolerate distractions while running a behavior support program or setting up a picture schedule, they will need to practice the skill a few times in situations that resemble those conditions. Trainers must remember that learners may be able to perform well in a classroom or a quiet office, but not perform those same skills when conditions are more difficult or complicated (Smith, Parker, Taubman, & Lovaas, 1992). This is especially true when staff members see themselves as being at risk.

Care providers are probably nervous and anxious about what to do in crisis situations and all the new things they need to learn. They may be afraid of injury, investigations, failure, embarrassment, or of not being adequately gifted to provide behavior support or handle a tough challenge. If frightened or nervous, they are not in a good "learning state." People learn best when they feel comfortable and safe. Trainers must consider what they can do to reduce the fear factor regarding the crisis and increase the confidence level of the trainees. The more positive an environment a trainer can create, the more likely the learner is to succeed (Jensen, 1995). A key component of the learning environment is created by language used in training. Technical jargon, while handy in communication among experienced practitioners, often is incomprehensible to care providers. Jargon use during training sessions should be minimized, and any technical language used must be explained clearly and "translated."

It is extremely important for learners to be involved in the training. People do not retain information well through passive learning experiences. This theme — of an active learning experience — holds across the range of learners (Engelmann & Carnine, 1991). Training should involve the new staff physically, mentally, and emotionally. Figure 9.1 depicts the level of retention for different types of learning experiences (Carr, 1992; Hart, 1991; McArdle, 1993; Reay, 1994). Through lecture alone, most people will remember a small amount of what is said. If they are involved in discussions and demonstrations, that retention rate increases. The highest rate of retention comes with immediate use or through teaching the material to somebody else.

Learning, as reflected in the performance of new or changed behaviors, is the desired outcome of training; many trainers see their job only as presenting information as quickly as possible, especially in reactive modes of consultation. If trainers quickly unload lots of information on the new staff (most of which is forgotten), they are really wasting, not saving, valuable time. Staff trainers must use methods of training that involve the learner more, even though such activities may be more time consuming. This will produce better results in the long run through increased competency, fewer errors, and less retraining (Acosta-Amad & Brethower, 1992; DuBois, 1993).

There are particular and specific training needs for improving staff performance in behavior support. First, the field is constantly evolving and changing. One need only look at recent changes in best-practice intervention for severe behavior problems, as described in this volume. Controversies remain, however. The continuing debate about use of aversive stimuli in behavior support remains an important issue and is frequently addressed in professional communication (Helmstetter & Durand, 1991; Repp & Singh, 1990; Thompson, 1990). This is an important topic to teach to care providers as well. Consultants may recommend the use of support strategies beyond the skill level of the care providers. Systems changes driven by self-determination may revolutionize the field of support (O'Brien, 1994; Sands & Wehmeyer, 1996). In a field in which best practices are evolving constantly, there is a significant need for training on new, emerging ideas (Mittler, 1987). Second, community-based systems are serving people who present more significant challenges, whether behavioral or medical. As the demographics of people supported in community settings change, the necessary staff

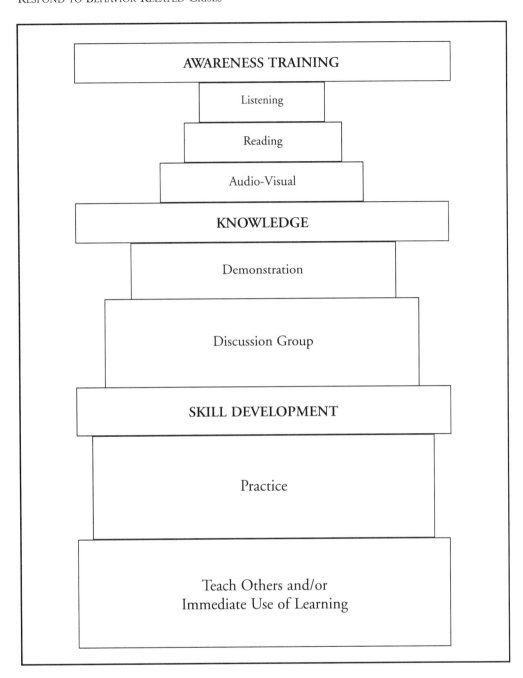

Figure 9.1. Range of retention for types of learning experiences.

skills change as well. Finally, demands for improvement to systems serving people with disabilities (e.g., advocacy and governmental regulations) also may change the requisite staff skills (Shapiro, 1994).

Training for care providers regarding positive behavior support typically includes a number of topics (Dunlap et al., 2000). Due to the comprehensive nature of positive behavior support, the specific topics chosen depend on the unique needs of the situation. Specific topics often are chosen initially by the consultant or trainer, with subsequent review and comment from the people who are to be trained and other stakeholders. Table 9.3 presents a list of topics.

TABLE 9.3
Topics for Training in Positive Behavior Support

- Values regarding positive behavior support

- Reasons why people with disabilities are more likely to have problem behaviors

- Knowledge specific to types of disability or mental illness (e.g., autism or borderline personality disorder)

- Creating positive environments

- Basic information regarding functional assessment

- How to participate in a functional assessment

- Data utility and collection strategies

- Data-based decision making

- Strategies for behavior support (e.g., functional communication training)

- Person-specific strategies (e.g., dos and don'ts with a person)

- Evaluation strategies for plan effectiveness

- Continuous quality improvement

- Team member issues and collaboration

- Physical intervention

- De-escalation

- Behavioral escalation

- Responding to setting event

Is Training Effective?

Although administrators of many residential providers may call for better staff training to ameliorate performance deficits (Bruininks, Kudla, Wieck, & Hauber, 1980; Burch, Reiss, & Bailey, 1987), studies spanning a range of years have demonstrated that standard training sessions alone often do not change targeted staff behaviors in an observable, significant fashion (e.g, Delameter, Connors, & Wells, 1984; Quilitch, 1975; Suda & Miltenberger, 1993). This does not mean that these training sessions were useless for promoting appropriate staff behavior; the studies only show that they were not sufficient (Reid, Parsons, & Green, 1989). Intuitively, both skills and motivation are necessary in maximizing direct care performance. Investigators have long recognized that failures to emit a targeted behavior may be due to one of two reasons. First, the individual may not know how to perform the behavior. Second, the individual may know how to perform the behavior, but may not have sufficient incentive to perform that behavior at appropriate times (Gresham, 1981). Examination of management structure and performance in social services must consider employee skill level in addition to motivation.

Existing training systems used in behavior support often are not sufficient. Pull-out systems are commonly used, yet data exist that show its inadequacy in changing staff performance (Smith et al., 1992). Train-the-trainer approaches hold promise, yet these are incumbent on the quality of internal trainers, which cannot be assumed and often is challenged. Baker and Feil (2000) documented that agency administrative staff reported that their agencies often do not have the capacity consistently to train or mentor new staff regarding behavior support. It is evident that new, comprehensive approaches are necessary in behavior support training as well as in other areas of training, going beyond traditional training methods, taking adult learning principles into account, and working in conjunction with local management (LaVigna, Willis, Shaull, Abedi, & Sweitzer, 1994).

Roles and Training of Management

Effective technical assistance and training efforts call for crucial supportive participation of local management. The first function is to support high-quality employee performance. Review of literature suggests the primary effective strategy may be ongoing feedback from the manager (Burgio & Burgio, 1990; Cullen, 1988). Although managerial feedback systems may be unfeasible for every desired staff behavior, other systems are documented to be effective (Hrydowy & Martin, 1994). Informal managerial feedback is more efficient than formal systems, but is less likely to be maintained as other pressing responsibilities arise. A formal system of performance review is desirable and documented to be effective in raising performance standards for behavior support as well as other areas (LaVigna et al.,

1994). The reader is referred to Burgio and Burgio (1990) and Cullen (1988) for more information and comprehensive reviews of literature.

Maintenance of employee morale is a second function of local management; this is likely to result in high performance, but is often difficult to achieve. Celebrating small victories is a helpful strategy, and continuously pointing out to staff members the progress, importance, and necessity of their work is helpful, especially in times of behavioral challenges (Arco, 1991).

A third function of local management during technical assistance efforts is to act as a liaison between the technical assistance provider and care providers. The manager can pass information from the care providers to the consultant, and pass suggestions from the technical assistance provider to the care providers. Without a single person acting as point of contact, information can be lost or misinterpreted (Foxx, 1996; Sprague et al., 1996).

We recommend specific strategies for consultants working in collaboration with local management. First, it is generally useful to include representatives from local management in all decisions. Teaching local management staff to work through decision-making processes will support their effective decision making in the future. Second, consultants should build an alliance with existing employee training systems. The consultant may recommend topics to include in the employee training, whether person-specific or generic. Third, the consultant can leave materials that may help in creating durable change in training for staff, for example, giving care providers written or electronic resources. The consultant also can point the care providers toward future resources.

Whereas the previous section focused on training issues for direct care providers, "line managers" (if applicable) represent an additional area of need in training. *Line manager* refers to a person who has at least partial responsibility for supervising direct care providers. Although this is unlikely to occur in family or foster settings, line managers are often found in agency-based supports. High-quality performance of managers is crucial to success to correct implementation of consultant recommendations. Table 9.4 lists topics that may be useful for managers and coordinators. The role of the consultant may or may not include technical assistance for management; that must be negotiated as part of the initial agreement. If the agreement does not include this category of technical assistance and training, but the consultant notes a problem in this area, it is appropriate for the consultant to request assistance or intervention from agency management or administration. Cooperation with local management can "make or break" the success of consultation (Baker, 1998; Foxx, 1996; Sulzer-Azaroff, Pollack, & Fleming, 1992).

TABLE 9.4
Topics for Manager Training

- Motivation of staff
- Behavioral support strategies
- Management of behavior programs
- Management in chaotic situations
- Assurance of staff performance
- Basics in case management
- Prioritization of tasks
- Work with behavioral consultants or specialists
- Continuous quality improvement
- Data collection and use

Proactive Strategies for Technical Assistance and Training

The best crisis intervention is one that prevents the crisis in the first place. Responding to crises creates significant tumult for all people involved as well as engendering significant financial strain. One person being in crisis can destabilize care providers, whether a family or an entire agency, and disrupt the lives of all around him or her. Training and technical assistance can play a significant part in reducing the threat of crisis. To achieve crisis prevention, agencies and care providers must have resources to provide assistance on an ongoing basis. As noted earlier, this could involve either training or technical assistance.

Identification of People Presenting Potential Risks

It is unlikely there will ever be sufficient resources to provide technical assistance to all people in the community. We recommend some sort of screening tool to help identify where resources are needed. Table 9.5 presents one form of screening, a risk matrix. The risk matrix was developed by a focus group in Oregon and notes the various types of behavioral and psychiatric risks that may be presented by individuals. A variation of this risk matrix will be used to assess the risks presented by people with disabilities receiving supports in Oregon. This risk matrix summarizes and presents concerns for an individual at a point in time. These levels of risk can change over time, and as the American Association on Mental Retardation definition of mental retardation points out, current functioning always needs to be seen as a balance of the individual and the environment (Luckasson et al., 1992). Risk can be created by the environment as well as by the individual. To prevent the misuse of this assessment, the following cautions must be exercised: (a) do not use the knowledge of risk to further stigmatize a person or justify more restrictive placement; (b) understand that past history does not mean that future recurrence of problem behavior is going to happen; (c) use the information to build capacity, not to demoralize care providers; and (d) corroborate interview or survey information with other sources of information as necessary.

TABLE 9.5
Behavioral and Mental Health Risk Factors

Part 1: Behavioral Risk Factors

Factor	High Risk	Medium Risk	Low Risk/NA
1. *Frequency of use of physical restraint due to behaviors dangerous to self or others*	Physical intervention is used monthly or more	Physical intervention used in last year but less frequently than monthly	Physical intervention last used more than 1 year ago or NA
2. *Intensity of aggressive or self-injurious acts (including pica)*	Caused injury which required medical attention within the last year	Caused injury in last year but no medical attention required	History of causing injury but more than a year ago or NA
3. *Escalation to aggression or self-injury*	Rapid escalation, no time to get assistance	Rapid escalation, but time to get assistance	Slow escalation, possible to prevent escalation or NA
4. *Rapid changes in frequency or intensity of behavior (across weeks or days)*	Rapid changes make it difficult to provide support for the person	Rapid changes, but currently do not create difficulties for care providers	No rapid changes in frequency or intensity or NA
5. *Property destruction resulting in injury to self or others*	Property destruction which resulted in need for medical attention within the last year	Property destruction which caused injury in last year but no medical attention required	History of property destruction which resulted in injury more than 1 year ago or NA

continued

Table 9.5, *continued*

Factor	High Risk	Medium Risk	Low Risk/NA
6. *Property destruction resulting in significant/substantial damage to homes, vehicles, or other properties*	Caused damage in the last year in excess of $100	Caused damage in the last year of a total of less than $100	History of property destruction more than 1 year ago or NA
7. *Fire-setting*	History of setting fires **or** fire-setting-related behaviors within last 5 years, such as collecting flammable objects	Comments regarding setting fires within last 5 years **or** history of fire-setting-related behavior less than 5 years ago	History of comments regarding setting fires more than 5 years ago or NA
8. *Inappropriate sexual behavior in community settings*	Has engaged in inappropriate sexual behaviors in community settings in the last 10 years	Has made comments or shown interest in last 10 years	History of inappropriate sexual behaviors more than 10 years ago or NA
9. *Targets others for predatory or victimizing sexual behavior*	Has targeted others in last 10 years	Has made comments or shown interest in last 10 years	History of targeting others more than 10 years ago or NA
10. *Attempts to leave home, work, or other settings without supervision or monitoring **and** is vulnerablee or unsafe in the community*	More than one incident in last year or one prolonged incident	One incident in last year of short duration	History of attempting to leave more than 1 year ago or NA
11. *Use of weapons to attempt to injure self or others*	Use of weapons in last 10 years	Has made comments or shown interest in last 10 years	History of weapon use more than 10 years ago or NA
12. *Engages in behaviors which result in community response or complaint*	More than one incident in last year	One incident in last year	History of causing community response or complaint more than 1 year ago or NA

continued

TABLE 9.5, *continued*

Part 2: Mental Health Risk Factors

Factor	High Risk	Medium Risk	Low Risk/NA
1. Actively searching for opportunities to harm self or others	More than 1 incident in last year or 1 prolonged incident (e.g., more than 1 week long)	One incident in last year	History more than 1 year ago or NA
2. Drug or alcohol problems	Currently experiencing drug or alcohol problems **and not** receiving or accepting treatment	Currently experiencing drug and alcohol problems **and** receiving treatment	History of drug or alcohol use, but not currently experiencing problems or NA
3. Mental health conditions or mental health diagnosis	Mental health condition resulting in significant disruption to life interfering with daily routine or relationships	Mental health condition in last year, but no disruption or interference with life	History of mental health conditions more than 1 year ago or NA
4. Cruelty to animals	Incident(s) of cruelty to animals in last 10 years	Has made comments or shown interest in last 10 years	History of cruelty more than 10 years ago or NA
5. Expressions of fantasies about hurting self or others, including suicide threats	One or more direct comments in last year	Shown interest in last year	History of comments more than 1 year ago or NA
6. Use of inpatient psychiatric care	More than one hospitalization in last year	One hospitalization in last year	History of hospitalization more than 1 year ago or NA

We recommend that behavior specialists use an assessment such as the risk matrix to identify people at higher risk of behavioral crisis. Once the appropriate population is identified, the factors that maintain appropriate behavior and stability of placement can be identified, and behavior support can occur in a proactive manner with the goal of preventing crisis and reactive modes of intervention.

Risk From Environments

It is important to recognize that behavioral risk factors and challenges interact with care provider and agency capacity. Baker and Feil (2000) described findings from a survey of 46 agencies providing support to people with disabilities. A set of 64 questions was asked regarding capacity to support people with disabilities who presented challenging behaviors. The 64 factors were organized into a set of two areas (ie., organizational stability and administrative leadership) considered to be independent measures and four areas (i.e., staff structures, staff training, measurement systems, behavioral systems) considered dependent measures. The measures were all highly intercorrelated, with administrative leadership most highly correlated with high levels of the three dependent measures, staff structures, measurement systems, and behavioral systems. Specific areas of low capacity were noted in all dependent measures, including features such as inadequate resources for behavior support (reported by 40% of all agencies). Insufficient resources have significant implications for success of consulting efforts (Foxx, 1996).

Site-specific concerns are also important to consider. It is recommended that consultants consider the capacity of the individual site or home as well as the agency. The Positive Environment Checklist (PEC) is one strategy to assess a site (Albin, Horner, & O'Neill, 1994). The PEC considers factors associated with the positive nature of a site, such as patterns of interaction, physical plant, and communication among people. A second set of considerations regard the relation between administrative features of the site and the high, median, or low risk of crisis intervention procedures (see Table 9.6).

With knowledge of the risk factors presented by an individual and the capacity of the care providers or agency, a behavior specialist is able to identify the people most likely to present some risk of crisis. The behavior specialist also is aware of the factors in the setting that help prevent crises or risk of further destabilization. With that information, the behavior specialist is able to tailor training or technical assistance strategies with the highest probabilities of success.

The reader is also encouraged to review the concerns presented previously regarding any such assessment of risk (see Table 9.5).

Possible Consultant Activities

In a proactive, or precrisis, mode a technical assistance provider is given leeway to work more slowly. Nondirective consultation, as described previously, becomes an option. In nondirective consultation, due to the greater involvement of team members, the team often learns new skills and abilities to use in future settings or situations. It is assumed, though, that a behavior specialist will often be able to write plans and move more quickly than other team members due to prior experience. In proactive technical assistance, the specialist can pay greater attention to team building and capacity raising, primarily using an instructional point of view

TABLE 9.6
Interaction Between Administration Features and Risk Potential

Factor	High Risk	Medium Risk	Low Risk/NA
1. *Difficulty implementing the behavior plan*	Few if any parts of the plan are being implemented	Some parts of the plan implemented	All parts of the plan implemented or NA
2. *Lack of training for family or staff in any area of support*	No training, but training is necessary	Some training, but more is needed	Training is sufficient or NA
3. *Difficulty in providing support due to factors such as burnout, lack of support, family or agency instability or burnout*	Difficulties present severe problems in providing support	Difficulties present some problems	Difficulties do not present problems or no difficulties or NA
4. *Care provider (family or staff) or team agreement regarding programmatic decisions or goals*	There is disagreement which results in problems for care providers (family or staff), such as failure to make decisions or refusal to work together	There is disagreement, but people still work together	Care providers make decisions smoothly and work together to resolve disagreement or NA
5. *Decision makers (family or agency staff) do not support person living in present environment*	Decision makers do not support person living in present home and think the person should not be there	Decision makers question person living in present home	Decision makers support person living in present home or NA
6. *Stability of home*	Home is unstable or person is homeless	Home is stable now, but may become unstable	Home is stable
7. *Fit with house mates or other people in house, including siblings*	Extensive problems between person and others escalating to problem behaviors, such as verbal or physical aggression	Some problems between person and others, but no escalation to problem behaviors	No problems between person and others or NA

with the team of care providers (see chap. 13, this volume).

In proactive modes, the consultant also may pay more attention to educating and working with local management. With the care provider or agency, the consultant can suggest systems change and improvement, because immediate attention is not focused on solving a crisis and maintaining placement and safety. In practice, though, these opportunities are not always present. Crises invariably will occur. The next section of this chapter covers reactive strategies.

Reactive Strategies for Training and Technical Assistance

As noted in the introduction of this chapter, when a crisis is occurring, the main focus of the care providers is on physical containment. People want to be trained in how to physically manage an individual who is presenting challenging behaviors, but this needs to be seen within the context of lifestyle issues. While physical intervention is sometimes necessary for the safety of the person and others, it must not be the sole topic of training and technical assistance. The focus of training and technical assistance should be the development of comprehensive behavior support plans. O'Neill et al. (1997) lists other topics in comprehensive behavior support plans as including strategies to address: (a) setting events, (b) antecedents to problem behavior, (c) skills deficits, (d) supporting appropriate behavior, (e) minimizing rewards for inappropriate behavior, and (f) addressing lifestyle issues.

A crisis prevention and intervention plan, with clearly described procedures for support providers, is an essential component of a comprehensive positive behavioral support plan for any person at risk of behavioral crisis (i.e., has a history of crisis or other high risk factors). Support providers should be trained to recognize early warning signs that behavioral escalation or crisis may occur. These signs may include indicator or "precursor" behaviors performed by the person with disability (e.g., increased arousal or agitation, low intensity problem behaviors that may escalate if not properly addressed). The presence of particular setting events in the physical environment (e.g., high levels of noise or confusion, disruption of typical schedules or routines) or in a person's "internal" environment (e.g., lack of sleep, physical pain or discomfort due to illness, allergy, or other physical condition) also may serve as "crisis alert" signs, because they may increase the probability of problem behaviors and escalation (Horner, Vaughn, Day, & Ard, 1996). Positive behavioral support plans should include neutralizing routines that can be implemented by support providers when relevant setting events are present (Horner, Day, & Day, 1997) and deescalation strategies that can be used when precursor behaviors or early signs of behavioral escalation are observed. A crisis plan also should provide a clear delineation of steps to be taken by support providers when indicators of a possible "blow-up" are present. These steps may include early notification of back-up support providers or implementation of procedures designed to reduce the likelihood of escalation (e.g., staff responses that are not confrontational) or to minimize the risk of harm (e.g., remove dangerous objects from a setting).

In reactive, crisis-driven technical assistance and training, speed of assistance is often critical. Training care providers on all aspects of behavior support is not always possible. We recommend that people be trained initially on person-specific rather than generic skills. More generic topics can be trained once the person-specific skills are developed. Competency-based training is a requirement to assure that care providers understand the new skills that are being trained (DuBois, 1993; Jensen, 1995). This includes positive skill-building types of intervention as well as physical intervention. Collaboration with management staff at the site of placement can assure that opportunities to practice these skills are created and receive managerial support. Especially in a rapid-response crisis situation, it is easy to simply train once and then move on, but this is to be avoided.

One aspect often overlooked is the emotional state of care providers during crisis situations. Clinicians often forget that the people implementing the plan need support themselves. While the specialist may not have the opportunity to provide direct support for all people involved, the clinician can model appropriate support. It is important that local management makes sure that the people providing support to the individual in crisis are acknowledged and appreciated. Clinicians can work with the local management to address problems in recruitment and retention in crisis situations, rather than simply treating turnover as a fait accompli. Strategies to improve recruitment and retention are being increasingly investigated in human services (Larson, Lakin, & Bruininks, 1998).

As a final note, in any crisis situation, emotions run strong and significant disagreements among team members are common. While the specialist should not get "in the middle" of any disagreement, the behavior specialist must always advocate for what is best for resolving the crisis. Negotiation is a very important skill in these situations, and win-win negotiation as described in the book *Getting to Yes* (Fisher & Ury, 1981) has been found very effective. Above all, in crisis situations the behavior specialist must model appropriate behavior, communication, and teamwork to achieve optimal outcomes.

Outcome Measures and Evaluation

The most common outcome measure for behavior support is an assessment of the frequency of problem behavior. Many excellent and thorough resources exist for further information on this topic (Johnston & Pennypacker, 1993). However, effective behavior support should do more than reduce problem behaviors. It should affect all aspects of a person's life, including one's overall health and safety, levels of adaptive skills, and quality of life (Horner et al., 1990; Horner, Close et al., 1996; Meyer & Janney, 1989). Common outcome measures in these situations include analyses of placement maintenance, measures of injuries or emergency health treatments (e.g., injury of people being restrained, lost work time injuries among people engaging in physical intervention), and measures of skill development (e.g., use of appropriate communication or other replacement behaviors). To achieve this goal, measures of an individual's lifestyle both prior and subsequent to the consultant's services are important. One method of achieving measures of lifestyle changes is operationally defining the critical parameters in the individual's life. These lifestyle measures can be transformed into statements and respondents can rate each statement on a Likert-type scale.

For example, questions may read:

• At this time, to what extent is this person socially integrated in the community?

• At this time, to what degree does this person have an opportunity to make choices?

• At this time, to what extent does the person have opportunities to participate in a variety of activities?

Each of the statements would be evaluated by the respondent by (a) never, (b) sometimes, (c) most of the time, (d) always. Ideally, 8 to 10 statements would be presented to the respondent.

The person conducting the ratings should be someone not involved in consultant supportive services for individual with disabilities. This will prevent bias in the respondents' ratings. An intake or referral person would be able to conduct this function face to face or over the phone as long as he or she is not directly involved in the care or service provision for the person with disabilities.

These statements would be presented to the person's case manager, the legally authorized representative, the person's primary caregiver and, if appropriate, the person receiving services. The person with disabilities must be able to respond to questions on a modified scale with short statements. In this case, the consultant would complete the scale with the person, even though in all other situations it would be a person external to direct involvement. The ideal time to take the first measure would be at the intake referral of the person in need of services. Phone or interpersonal contacts for the individual completion of the questionnaire by the case manager, legally authorized representative, and primary support caregiver would be made. Each will be asked to provide the ratings corresponding to the 2 weeks prior to initiation of consultation. The next ratings will be at the completion of the consultant's support services or once implementation of new strategies is up and running.

Another rating will be completed 4 months following the prior data point. This measure of the durability of lifestyle changes is important. The information obtained from these follow-up ratings may be useful for the interdisciplinary team's judgment if additional consultant services are needed.

For each of these measures, it is critical the same respondent provides rating both prior to and after services. For example, if the case manager changes, subsequent ratings will be useful minimally in the evaluation of changes. Once the initial ratings and the ratings obtained after the completion of services are obtained for a number of consumers, inferential statistical analyses can be conducted; that is, the ratings on each item will be statistically compared. For example, if the item reads, "At this time, to what extent is the person socially integrated in community?" the ratings on this item before and after consultant services would be statistically compared. Similar rating will be completed for all the other items. Likewise, the ratings obtained at the 4-month follow-up data point would be statistically compared to the ratings obtained prior to the initiation of services. Because the data obtained are ordinal, standard parametric statistical analyses would not be appropriate. However, the Wilcoxon matched-pairs signed-ranks is a nonparametric statistical test for related samples with only slightly less the power of a parametric analysis (Siegel, 1956). This test will analyze not only the direction of change, but also the magnitude of change.

Lifestyle measures for either individual consumers or a number of consumers receiving positive behavioral support services are important. Not only does the person benefit from objective measures of lifestyle enhancement, but consultants providing training and technical assistance services can critically evaluate their successes and areas on which improvement are needed.

Continuous improvement of behavior support plans is critical. Plans often need adjustment once they are implemented; the adjustment may involve fine tuning or wholesale retooling. Even if a plan is conceived correctly on the first try, modifications may be necessary once the person shows positive change. Each part of the plan should be reviewed through a regular quality improvement cycle; that is, each section should be considered with the process depicted in Figure 9.2, in

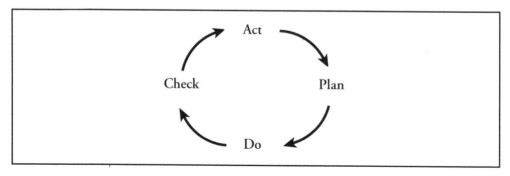

Figure 9.2. Quality Improvement Cycle.

which effectiveness of individual components is reviewed and adapted accordingly. A plan is developed, then implemented ("do"), then evaluated ("check"), then revised based on the evaluation ("act") (Shewhart, 1939).

Baker, Dean, and Sprague (1997) provide a more complete discussion of the use of continuous quality assurance in behavior consultation. If specific areas of the plan are not working, they should be revised with as much team input as is possible. Of particular note are any injuries or challenges to health and safety.

Summary

This chapter has presented considerations in training, technical assistance, and consultation in the prevention and response to challenging behavior and crisis situations. Consultants are in a unique role and play a crucial part in the effort to support people with disabilities in community settings. Recommendations have been given regarding models for technical assistance and best practices in training. Potential topics for training were listed, and suggestions were given for working with care providers and management staff. While all of these topics are important, ultimately the most important may be the degree of effectiveness in collaboration with care providers, a topic often ignored in the literature base. The authors hope to have added to this important area of service efficacy.

Author Note

Preparation of this chapter was supported in part by U.S. Department of Health and Human Services Grant No. 90DD0439 and U.S. Department of Education Grant No. H133B20004. However, the opinions expressed herein are those of the authors, and do not necessarily reflect the positions or policies of the governmental departments.

References

Acosta-Amad, S., & Brethower, D. M. (1992). Training for impact: Improving the quality of staff's performance. *Performance Improvement Quality, 5,* 2–13.

Albin, J. M. (1992). *Quality improvement in employment and other human services: Managing quality through change.* Baltimore: Paul H. Brookes.

Albin, J. M., Buckley, D., & Lynch, B. (1992). *Inservice preparation and presentation.* Specialized Training Program, University of Oregon.

Albin, R. W., Horner, R. H., & O'Neill, R. E. (1994). Proactive behavioral support: Structuring and assessing environments. Eugene: Rehabilitation Research and Training Center on Positive Behavioral Support, University of Oregon.

Arco, L. (1991). Effects of outcome performance feedback on maintenance of client and staff behavior in a residential setting. *Behavior Residential Treatment, 6,* 231–247.

Arco, L., & Birnbrauer, J. S. (1990). Performance feedback and maintenance of staff behavior in residential settings. *Behavioral Residential Treatment, 5*(3), 207–217.

Baker, D. J. (1998). Outcomes of behavior support training to an agency providing residential and vocational support to persons with disabilities. *Journal of The Association for Persons With Severe Handicaps, 23,* 144–148.

Baker, D. J., Dean, J., & Sprague, J. S. (1997). Continuous quality improvement applications in behavioral consultation. *Behavior Therapist, 20,* 121–125.

Baker, D. J., & Feil, E. (2000). A self-evaluation by agencies providing residential support of their capacity to support persons with disabilities and challenging behaviors. *International Journal of Disability, Development, and Education, 47,* 171–181.

Braddock, D., & Mitchell, D. (1992). *Residential services and developmental disabilities in the United States: A national survey of staff turnover, compensation, and related issues.* Washington, DC: American Association on Mental Retardation.

Bruininks, R. H., Kudla, M. J., Wieck, C. A., & Hauber, F. A. (1980). Management problems in community residential facilities. *Mental Retardation, 18,* 125–130.

Burch, M. R., Reiss, M. L., & Bailey, J. S. (1987). A competency-based "hands-on" training package for direct-care staff. *Journal of The Association for Persons With Severe Handicaps, 12,* 67–71.

Burgio, L., & Burgio, K. (1990). Institutional staff training and management: A review of the literature and a model for geriatric long-term care facilities. *International Journal of Aging and Human Development, 30*(4), 287–302.

Carr, C. (1992). *Smart training.* New York: McGraw Hill.

Cullen, C. (1988). A review of staff training: The emperor's old clothes. *Irish Journal of Psychology, 9*(2), 309–323.

Delameter, A. M., Connors, C. K., & Wells, K. C. (1984). A comparison of staff training procedures: Behavioral applications in the child psychiatric inpatient setting. *Behavioral Modification, 8,* 39–58.

Deming, W. E. (1986). *Out of the crisis.* Cambridge: Massachusetts Institute of Technology.

DuBois, D. D. (1993). *Competency-based performance measurement.* Amherst, MA: HRD.

Dunlap, G., Hieneman, M., Knoster, T., Fox, L., Anderson, J., & Albin, R. (2000). Essential elements of inservice training in positive behavior support. *Journal of Positive Behavior Interventions, 2,* 22–32.

Engelmann, S., & Carnine, D. (1991). *Theory of instruction: Principles and applications* (rev. ed.). Eugene, OR: ADI Press.

Fisher, R., & Ury, W. (1981). *Getting to yes.* Boston: Houghton Mifflin.

Foxx, R. M. (1996). Twenty years of applied behavior analysis in treating the most severe problem behaviors: Lessons learned. *The Behavior Analyst, 19,* 225–236.

Gresham, F. M. (1981). Social skills training with handicapped children: A review. *Review of Educational Research, 51,* 139–176.

Hart, L. B. (1991). *Training methods that work.* Menlo Park, CA: Crisp.

Helmstetter, E., & Durand, V. M. (1991). Nonaversive interventions for severe behavior problems. In L. H. Meyer, C. A. Peck, & L. Brown (Eds.), *Critical issues in the lives of people with severe disabilities* (pp. 559–600). Baltimore: Paul H. Brookes.

Horner, R. H. (1994). Functional assessment: Contributions and future directions. *Journal of Applied Behavior Analysis, 27*(2), 401–404.

Horner, R. H. (1999a). Positive behavior supports. In M. L. Wehmeyer & J. R. Patton (Eds.), *Mental retardation in the 21st century* (pp. 181–196). Austin, TX: Pro-Ed.

Horner, R. H., Albin, R. W., Sprague, J. R., & Todd, A. W. (1999b). Positive behavior support. In M. E. Snell & F. Brown (Eds.), *Instruction of students with severe disabilities* (5th ed.) (pp. 207–244). Upper Saddle River, NJ: Prentice Hall.

Horner, R. H., Close, D. W., Fredericks, H. D. (Bud), O'Neill, R. E., Albin, R. W., Sprague, J. R., Kennedy, C. H., Flannery, K. B., & Heathfield, L. T. (1996). Supported living for people with profound disabilities and severe problem behaviors. In D. H. Lehr & F. Brown (Eds.), *People with disabilities who challenge the system* (pp. 209–240). Baltimore: Paul H. Brookes.

Horner, R. H., Day, H. M., & Day, J. R. (1997). Using neutralizing routines to reduce problem behaviors. *Journal of Applied Behavior Analysis, 30,* 601–614.

Horner, R. H., Day, H. M., Sprague, J. R., O'Brien, M., & Heathfield, L. T. (1991). Interspersed requests: A nonaversive procedure for reducing aggression and self-injury during instruction. *Journal of Applied Behavior Analysis, 24,* 265–278.

Horner, R. H., Dunlap, G., Koegel, R. L., Carr, E. G, Sailor, W., Anderson, J., Albin, R. W., & O'Neill, R. E. (1990). Toward a technology of "nonaversive" behavioral support. *Journal of The Association for Persons With Severe Handicaps, 15,* 125–132.

Horner, R. H., Vaughn, B. J., Day, H. M., & Ard, W. R. (1996). The relationship between setting events and problem behavior: Expanding our understanding of behavioral support. In L. K. Koegel, R. L. Koegel, & G. Dunlap (Eds.), *Positive behavioral support: Including people with difficult behavior in the community* (pp. 381–402). Baltimore: Paul H. Brookes.

Hughes, J. N., & DeForest, P. A. (1993). Consultant directiveness and support as predictors of consultation outcomes. *Journal of School Psychology, 31,* 355–373.

Hrydowy, E. R., & Martin, G. L. (1994). A practical staff management package for use in a training program for persons with developmental disabilities. *Behavior Modification, 18*(1), 66–88.

Jensen, E. (1995). *Superteaching.* Del Mar, CA: Turning Point.

Johnston, J. M., & Pennypacker, H. S. (1993). *Strategies and tactics of behavioral research.* Hillsdale, NJ: Lawrence Erlbaum.

Kratochwill, T. R., & Bergen, J. R. (1990). *Behavior Consultation in Applied Settings.* New York: Plenum.

Larson, S., Hewitt, A., & Lakin, K. C. (1994). Residential Services Personnel. In B. H. Abery & M. F. Hayden (Eds.), *Challenges for a service system in transition: Ensuring quality community experiences for persons with developmental disabilities* (pp. 313–341). Baltimore: Paul H. Brookes.

Larson, S. A., Lakin, K. C., & Bruininks, R. H. (1998). *Staff recruitment and retention: Study results and intervention strategies.* Washington, DC: American Association on Mental Retardation.

LaVigna, G. W., Willis, T. J., Shaull, J. F., Abedi, M., & Sweitzer, M. (1994). *Periodic service review: A total quality assurance system for human services and education.* Baltimore: Paul H. Brookes.

Luckasson, R., Coulter, D. L., Polloway, E. A., Reiss, S., Schalock, R. L., Snell, M. E., Spitalnik, D. M., & Stark, J. A. (1992). *Mental retardation: Definition, classification, and systems of support.* Washington, DC: American Association on Mental Retardation.

Lucyshyn, J. M., & Albin, R. W. (1993). Comprehensive support to families of children with disabilities and behavior problems: Keeping it "friendly." In G. H. S. Singer & L. E. Powers (Eds.), *Families, disability, and empowerment: Active coping skills and strategies for family interventions* (pp. 365–407). Baltimore: Paul H. Brookes.

Mace, F. C. (1994). The significance and future of functional analysis methodologies. *Journal of Applied Behavior Analysis, 27,* 385–392.

Mace, F. C., Hock, M. L., Lalli, J. S., West, B. J., Belfiore, P., Pinter, E., & Brown, D. K. (1988). Behavioral momentum in the treatment of noncompliance. *Journal of Applied Behavior Analysis, 21,* 123–141.

McArdle, G. E. H. (1993). *Delivering effective training sessions.* Menlo Park, CA: Crisp.

Meyer, L. H., & Janney, R. E. (1989). User-friendly measures of meaningful outcomes: Evaluating behavioral interventions. *Journal of The Association for Persons With Severe Handicaps, 14,* 263–270.

Mittler, P. J. (1987). Staff development: Changing needs and service contexts in Britain. In J. Hogg & P. Mittler (Eds.), *Staff training in mental handicap.* Beckenham, UK: Croom Helm.

O'Brien, J. (1994). Down stairs that are never your own: Supporting people with developmental disabilities in their own homes. *Mental Retardation, 32*(1), 1–6.

O'Neill, R. E., Horner, R. H., Albin, R. W., Sprague, J. R., Storey, K., & Newton, J. S. (1997). *Functional assessment and program development for problem behavior: A practical handbook* (2nd ed.). Pacific Grove, CA: Brooks/Cole.

Quilitch, H. R. (1975). A comparison of three staff-management procedures. *Journal of Applied Behavior Analysis, 8,* 59–66.

Reay, D. G. (1994). *Selecting training methods.* East Brunswick, NJ: Nichols.

Reid, D. H., Parsons, M. B., & Green, C. W. (1989). *Staff management in human services.* Springfield, IL: Charles C. Thomas.

Repp, A. C. (1999). Naturalistic functional assessment with regular and special education students in classroom settings. In A. C. Repp & R. H. Horner (Eds.), *Functional analysis of problem behavior: From effective assessment to effective support* (pp. 238–258). Belmont, CA: Wadsworth.

Repp, A. C., & Singh, N. N. (1990). *Perspectives on the use of nonaversive and aversive interventions for persons with developmental disabilities.* Sycamore, IL: Sycamore.

Rudolph, C., Lakin, K. C., Oslund, J. M., & Larson, W. (1998). Evaluation of outcomes and cost-effectiveness of a community behavioral support and crisis response demonstration project. *Mental Retardation, 36,* 187–197.

Rule, S., Fodor-Davis, J., Morgan, R., Salzberg, C. L., & Chen, J. (1990). An in-service training model to encourage collaborative consultation. *Teacher Education and Special Education, 13*(3), 225–227.

Sands, D. J., & Wehmeyer, M. L. (1996). *Self-determination across the life span: Independence and choice for people with disabilities.* Baltimore: Paul H. Brookes.

Shapiro, J. P. (1994). How the parents of disabled kids are shaking up the nation. *U.S. News and World Report, 116*(1), 38–42.

Shewhart, W. A. (1939). Statistical methods from the viewpoint of quality control. Washington, DC: U.S. Department of Agriculture.

Shores, R. E., Wehby, J. H., & Jack, S. L. (1999). Analyzing behavior disorders in classrooms. In A. C. Repp & R. H. Horner (Eds.), *Functional analysis of problem behavior: From effective assessment to effective support* (pp. 219–237). Belmont, CA: Wadsworth.

Siegel, S. (1956). *Nonparametric statistics for the behavioral sciences.* New York: McGraw-Hill.

Smith, T., Parker, T., Taubman, M., & Lovaas, O. I. (1992). Transfer of staff training from workshops to group homes: A failure to generalize across settings. *Research in Developmental Disabilities, 13,* 57–72.

Snell, M. (1990). Building our capacity to meet the needs of persons with severe disabilities. In A. P. Kaiser & C. M. McWhorter (Eds.), *Preparing personnel to work with persons with severe disabilities.* Baltimore: Paul H. Brookes.

Sprague, J. R., Flannery, B., O'Neill, R., & Baker, D. J. (1996). *Effective behavioral consultation: Supporting the implementation of positive behavior support plans for persons with severe problem behaviors.* Eugene, OR: Specialized Training Program.

Suda, K., & Miltenberger, R. (1993). Evaluation of staff management strategies to increase positive interactions in a vocational setting. *Behavioral Residential Treatment, 8,* 69–88.

Sulzer-Azaroff, B., Pollack, M. J., & Fleming, R. K. (1992). Organizational behavior management within structural and cultural constraints: An example from the human service sector. *Journal of Organizational Behavior Management, 12,* 117–137.

Thompson, T. (1990). The humpty dumpty world of aversive interventions. *Journal of The Association for Persons With Severe Handicaps, 15,* 136–139.

Wlodkowski, R. (1985). *Enhancing adult motivation to learn.* San Francisco, CA: Jossey-Bass.

CHAPTER 10

Using Functional Assessment and Systems-Level Assessment to Build Effective Behavioral Support Plans

Rachel Freeman
University of Kansas
Lawrence, Kansas

Daniel Baker
Oregon Rehabilitation Association
Salem, Oregon

Robert Horner
University of Oregon
Eugene, Oregon

Chris Smith
Jody Britten
Amy McCart
University of Oregon
Eugene, Oregon

Functional assessment is an integral part of positive behavioral support (Koegel, Koegel, & Dunlap, 1996). Information gathered in a functional assessment identifies the variables that predict and maintain problem behavior. This information is used to improve the effectiveness and efficiency of behavioral support plans

(Carr, Langdon, & Yarbrough, 1999). In some cases a functional assessment is necessary to support a person whose behavior has become so intense as to result in health or safety risks. The functional assessment process helps service providers build behavioral support plans that are technically sound in their application of behavioral principles.

An equally important task in positive behavioral support, however, is to gather information that takes into consideration people and environments in which the behavioral support plan will be implemented (Albin, Lucyshyn, Horner, & Flannery, 1996; McClannahan & Krantz, 1993). Once a functional assessment is complete, interventions that fit the resources, skills, and values of the individuals implementing the plan are needed (Horner, 1994). Failure to consider the systemic issues related to resource availability and the characteristics of individuals involved may result in inconsistent implementation or complete rejection of the behavioral support plan (Albin et al., 1996).

There is a significant amount of information available describing how functional assessment should be conducted ("Functional analysis approaches," 1994; O'Neill et al., 1997). Less effort, however, has been devoted to describing how functional assessment information is used to build and implement effective behavioral support plans (Horner, 1994). A critical element in the design and implementation of a behavioral support plan involves collaborative problem solving by those supporting an individual with problem behavior and systems-level changes within the environment. The attention paid to systemic variables related to behavioral support plan implementation can increase intervention effectiveness (McClannahan & Krantz, 1993). The purpose of this chapter is to: (a) describe how functional assessment fits within the larger context of behavioral support plan development, (b) discuss how assessment of systems-level variables contributes to the design and implementation of a behavioral support plan, and (c) explore issues related to functional assessment and systems-level assessment when an individual is engaging in such severe problem behavior that the person is described as being in a "crisis."

Functional Assessment

Functional assessment refers to a process for gathering information about an individual's behavior and environmental variables that influence that behavior (Foster-Johnson & Dunlap, 1993). A primary goal of functional assessment is to identify the function that maintains problem behavior (Horner & Carr, 1997). Behaviors are not repeated over time unless they are associated with a maintaining consequence: a function. Although there are a number of functions that may maintain problem behavior, they can be combined to form two major categories: to avoid or escape from something unpleasant or to obtain something desirable (O'Neill et al., 1997; Reichle & Johnston, 1993).

Problem behavior may occur when an individual is trying to escape from an unpleasant situation (Carr & Newsom, 1985; Iwata, Pace et al., 1994). For example, a woman who dislikes shopping may throw chairs across the room because she knows that she will be told that she has to stay home. Problem behavior may also occur in order to avoid specific people, or to escape internal stimulation such as physical pain or illness (Carr & Smith, 1995; Taylor & Carr, 1992a, 1992b).

Some individuals engage in problem behavior to gain attention from their staff, teachers, family, or peers. In other cases problem behavior may serve to obtain preferred items or events (Derby et al., 1992; Durand & Crimmins, 1988). An individual's problem behavior can also be maintained by internal stimulation, as is the case when a person repetitively engages in a behavior to obtain sensory or tactile stimulation (Favell, McGimsey, & Schell, 1982; Koegel & Koegel, 1989).

Functional assessment methods also identify the variables that can be used to reliably predict problem behavior. Antecedents are events that immediately precede the occurrence of problem behavior. Demands, critical feedback, or the types of tasks presented to an individual are all examples of antecedents that may evoke problem behavior. Setting events are broader contextual variables that increase the likelihood that an antecedent cue will trigger problem behavior (Carr, Reeve, & Magito-McLaughlin, 1996). Research indicates that setting events can be due to environmental, social, or physiological factors (Brown, 1991; Carr & Smith, 1995; Dadson & Horner, 1993; Horner, 1980; Horner, Vaughn, Day, & Ard, 1996). Environmental setting events may occur when a student's routine is disrupted and he or she is unable to predict upcoming events. Social setting events may include being left alone for a period of time or fighting with a family member or roommate. Illness, pain, sleep deprivation, hunger, and medication changes are just a few examples of internal factors that increase the likelihood of problem behaviors.

Characteristics of Functional Assessment

The major focus of functional assessment is to gather information that will be used to redesign the environment rather than trying to "fix" or "change" an individual. It is important to remember that problem behavior does not occur in a vacuum; it occurs within a social network or system (Carr, Langdon, & Yarbrough, 1994). To support an individual who engages in problem behavior, we must often consider the interaction between the individual and at least one other person. The responsibility for change is shared by those concerned with the individual's problem behavior. Teaching an individual new skills requires family or support staff to create opportunities for these skills to be used and respond accordingly. Even when problem behaviors are maintained by physiological events such as the presence of illness or pain, how other individuals respond within the social network may have an impact on whether the behaviors escalate in intensity. The functional assessment process provides information about the social network that can be used to design effective behavioral support strategies. Understanding the strengths, preferences, and values within the social network increases the likelihood that a behavioral support plan will be a good "fit" for those involved in implementing the plans (Albin et al., 1996).

The situations and experiences encountered by individuals in one environment can naturally carry over into other settings where they live and socialize. For instance, a teacher may discover a student consistently engages in problem behaviors when the student hasn't had enough sleep the night before. Therefore, functional assessment information should take into consideration the individual's life across home, school, and work environments (Freeman et al., 1999).

A functional assessment allows one to gain information needed to improve the quality of life for both the individual engaging in problem behavior and for that person's entire social network. Functional assessment information provides a wider range of options within the community to individuals who engage in severe problem behavior (Guess, Helmstetter, Turnbull, & Knowlton, 1986; Horner, Sprague, & Flannery, 1993; Meyer & Evans, 1989; Turnbull & Guess, 1986). Strategies for improving quality of life may be more effective in reducing challenging behaviors than focusing on problem behavior alone (McGee, 1996). A variety of functional assessment methods can be used to gather information regarding the individual and his or her social network.

Functional Assessment Methods

Three types of functional assessment methods help to identify the function of a problem behavior: indirect assessment, direct assessment, and functional analysis. The number of methods you choose and the complexity of the functional assessment depend upon the needs of the individual and complexity of the situation. This section will provide a brief summary of functional assessment.

Indirect Assessment

Indirect assessment information is gathered by conducting interviews, reviewing written records, and using checklists and questionnaires (Drager et al., 1998). Interviews with key people are often an initial step used to determine the concerns regarding an individual's problem behavior. Interviews also can help identify and narrow the range of variables influencing the behavior (O'Neill et al., 1997). Individuals interviewed should include people present when problem behavior occurs or those who know the person well. The individual engaging in problem behavior may also be interviewed, although this varies depending upon communication skills and interest levels (Lewis-Palmer, Sugai, & Horner, 1999).

Record reviews provide information on past history, and quality-of-life measures highlight social aspects of the individual's life that may need attention.

Finally, using available checklists and rating scales provide insight into the function of the individual's problem behavior or the factors that may predict problem behavior (Durand, 1988, 1990).

Direct Assessment

Direct methods of assessment involve observing the individual to clearly identify when problem behavior occurs, what happens right before problem behavior, what problem behavior looks like, and how people respond to the occurrence of problem behavior. Many types of direct observation methods are available. Measurement methods can document the frequency, duration, latency, and intensity of problem behavior. An interval recording method, the scatter plot, is frequently used as a functional assessment documentation tool (O'Neill et al., 1997; Touchette, MacDonald, & Langer, 1985). Data are collected during specific time intervals across the day, allowing one to identify whether problem behaviors occur at predictable time periods. Narrative data can be collected to help identify and confirm the immediate events in the environment that precede and follow the occurrence of problem behavior (Bijou, Peterson, & Ault, 1968; Doss & Reichle, 1989; Touchette, MacDonald, & Langer, 1985). A descriptive method of data collection may involve documentation of identified setting events, antecedents, and maintaining consequences. Functional analysis, another functional assessment method, provides a way to empirically test your hypothesis.

Functional Analysis

A functional analysis systematically tests hypotheses by manipulating the variables or events that are thought to be associated with the occurrence of problem behavior (Horner, 1994; Horner & Carr, 1997; Iwata, Dorsey, Slifer, Bauman, & Richman, 1994). A functional analysis is a formal test of the relationship between environmental variables and the occurrence and nonoccurrence of problem behaviors. Each variable suspected to contribute to the occurrence of a problem behavior is isolated and presented in the absence of other competing sources of variance. Researchers often use this approach because it is the most precise and controlled method for demonstrating the functional relationship between environmental events and problem behavior (O'Neill et al., 1997).

A functional analysis may involve the manipulation of antecedent variables or consequences (Drager et al., 1998; O'Neill et al., 1997) although a combination of the two approaches can sometimes be used. Examples of antecedent variables that may be systematically introduced and withdrawn during functional analysis conditions include: attention from another person, certain activities or events, or specific instructions or tasks. These conditions may be designed to test whether an individual engages in problem behavior to gain attention; escape from tasks, people, or activities; obtain items; or obtain sensory stimulation (O'Neill et al., 1997).

A number of procedural approaches have been reported in the functional analysis literature. The extent to which the functional analysis simulates the individual's natural environment is an important consideration (Carr, Langdon, & Yarbrough, 1999). A major challenge is to design analogue settings that accurately reflect the actual conditions occurring within the natural environment and to sample all of the variables that may be contributing to the occurrence of problem behavior (Carr, Langdon, & Yarbrough, 1999). Indirect and direct functional assessment methods are often used to generate the information needed to design the functional analysis analogue conditions.

Outcomes of Functional Assessment

Any combination of functional assessment methods may be appropriate, depending on the individual's needs and the complexity of the situation (Tilly et al., 1998). The functional assessment process, however, remains the same whether a problem behavior is mild or severe in nature.

A functional assessment is considered complete when the following outcomes are accomplished: (a) there is a clear and measurable definition of the problem behavior, (b) the events, times, and situations that predict both the occurrence and nonoccurrence of problem behavior are determined, (c) consequences that maintain problem behavior are identified, (d) one or more hypotheses regarding the function maintaining problem behavior are developed, and (e) direct observation data identifying and confirming the function of the problem behavior is complete (O'Neill et al., 1997).

A functional assessment should provide information leading to behavioral support plans that address the function of an individual's problem behavior (see Figure 10.1). This usually involves multiple intervention strategies to address problem behavior in all of the routines and settings where it occurs. Multicomponent interventions may include manipulating antecedent or setting event variables, teaching new skills, manipulating consequences, and crisis intervention (Horner, Albin, & O'Neill, 1991; Horner, O'Neill, & Flannery, 1993; Lucyshyn & Albin, 1993).

Building Effective Behavioral Support Plans

Designing a Plan of Support

Once the functional assessment is completed, the next step is to design a behavioral support plan based on the information gathered (see Figure 10.2).

Information gathered from the functional assessment is used to design a

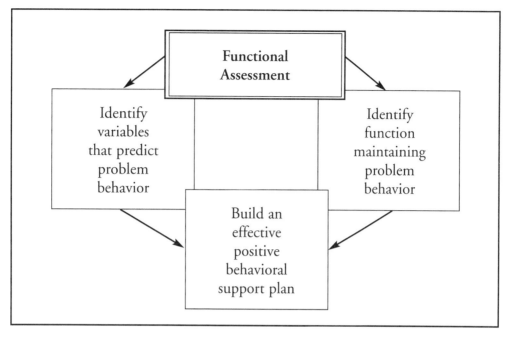

Figure 10.1. Functional assessment model.

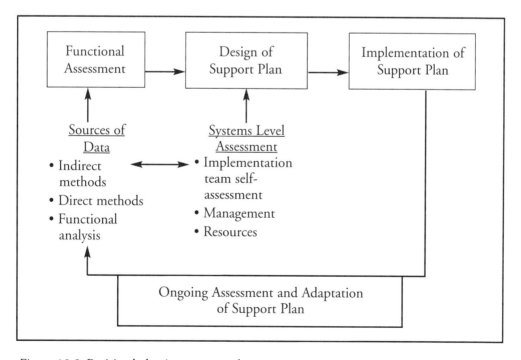

Figure 10.2. Positive behavior support plan process.

competing-behavior analysis (Horner, O'Neill, & Flannery, 1993; O'Neill et al., 1997). A competing behavior is one that has similar functional properties as the problem behavior. A competing-behavior analysis (CBA) helps the implementation team organize functional assessment information and identify key intervention strategies that will directly address the setting events, antecedents, and consequences that maintain problem behavior. The CBA goes a further step, including desired behaviors that an individual should be exhibiting and possible alternative behaviors meant to replace problem behavior. Using this approach one can identify logically linked interventions designed to replace problem behavior (i.e., teaching and reinforcing more socially appropriate behaviors). Figure 10.3 shows a competing-behavior analysis for a man named Sam. This part of the design process helps the implementation team create technically sound intervention plans.

In planning a support plan it is also important to pay attention to variables that will increase the contextual fit between the behavioral support plan and the implementation team. Many behavioral support plans that are technically sound are poorly implemented, not maintained over time, or filed away without ever being used (Albin et al., 1996). Implementation failure may be related to the lack of attention paid to whether or not a behavioral support plan matches the values, skills, and resources of the social network (Horner et al., 1996; Lucyshyn, Olson, & Horner, 1995). For instance, a behavior support plan with good contextual fit will (a) include interventions that work well in the target environment, (b) identify extra training for staff when needed, and (c) seek out resources available for behavioral support plan development. The involvement of the people who will be implementing the plan is essential to assure contextual fit. Important considerations involved in assessing both the technical soundness and contextual fit of a behavioral support plan can be found in the checklist in Table 10.1.

Implementing a Support Plan

Once the implementation team has decided upon the design of the behavioral support plan, the implementation process begins. Training needed to ensure a successful behavioral support plan begins during the implementation process. In addition, longitudinal strategies are needed to document the training process and information needed to introduce new members of the social network to the behavioral support plan.

Implementation also includes (a) establishing ongoing data collection systems, (b) setting up access to needed resources, and (c) creating administrative systems necessary for assuring fidelity of the behavioral support plan. For example, an administrative system may be designed so that staff are free to attend regular team meetings, review the data and make modifications to the plan, and embed the behavioral support plan training into larger staff development systems within an agency.

| Setting Event:
Change in work schedule | Antecedent:
No attention | Desired Behavior:
Working by himself or with peers

Problem Behavior:
Pulling hair

Replacement Behavior:
Requesting attention | Maintaining Consequences:
Staff praise after a designated time period or immediate attention from staff |

Logically linked intervention strategies addressing:

Setting-Event Interventions	Antecedent Interventions	Teaching New Skills	Consequence Interventions
• Obtain information from work site regarding changes in Sam's daily schedule given in advance • Conduct visual schedule and rehearsals with Sam	• Provide higher levels of attention during tough periods (setting events, higher levels of agitation, etc.)	• Teach Sam to request attention from staff • Teach Sam to gradually tolerate longer periods of time without staff attention • Teach Sam to build rapport with peers • Teach Sam how to initiate positive social interaction with both staff and peers	• Minimize the attention Sam gets when he engages in problem behavior • When possible, intervene before Sam pulls hair by redirecting when early warning signs appear (i.e., agitation, flapping or waving hands, both hands in front of his face, loud vocalizations) • Provide frequent praise for appropriate behavior

Adapted from *Functional Assessment and Program Development for Problem Behavior: A Practical Handbook* (2nd ed., p. 75), by R. E. O'Neill, R. H. Horner, R. W. Albin, J. R. Sprague, K. Storey, and J. S. Newton, Pacific Grove, CA: Brooks/Cole. Copyright 1997 by Brooks/Cole Publishing Company. Adapted with permission.

Figure 10.3. Designing a competing-behavior analysis.

TABLE 10.1
Checklist for the Behavioral Support Plan

Is the Plan Technically Sound?

1. Has a functional assessment been conducted?

2. Is there agreement on the daily routines where problems are most likely to occur?

3. Have operational definitions of the problem behaviors, and the events that reliably predict and maintain problem behaviors been identified?

4. Have the functional assessment hypotheses been used to define key features of an effective plan of support?

5. Does the plan have a clear and practical system for measuring success on an ongoing basis?

Is the Plan Contextually Sound?

1. Has the implementation team been involved in the plan's development?

2. Does the plan clearly define what is being done to make the environment different?

3. Are the procedures in the plan achievable given the skills people have?

4. Are people willing to implement the procedures? Are these procedures culturally appropriate?

5. Does the implementation team believe the procedures will be effective? Are the procedures in the best interest of the focus person?

6. Are the resources and materials needed to implement the plan available?

7. Is there observable administrative support for the plan? Is that support available to: provide adequate training, allocate time for staff participation, and allocate time to review and maintain the plan?

Ongoing Assessment and Adaptation

Once a behavior support plan is in place, some assume that further assessment is not needed. However, problem behavior is not static; in fact, it can change significantly over time. The people in an individual's social network may change, or the individual may move to a different home or community. Therefore, it is important to view functional assessment as an ongoing process, not a one-time event

(Horner, 1994). The functional assessment allows us to continually improve the behavioral support plan and assess resources that are needed to maintain a high quality of life for the individual and the entire social network.

Systems-Level Assessment

A systems-level assessment provides the implementation team with important information needed to ensure contextual fit. Building and implementing a positive behavioral support plan can be an empowering process for an implementation team. Following the guidelines (see Table 10.1) for assessing a behavioral support plan by addressing technical soundness and contextual fit may increase the effectiveness of the plan. In many cases the process for designing and assessing a behavioral support plan can easily take place as the team comes to consensus on various decisions that must be made. Sometimes, however, implementation team members may have diverse opinions and values, resulting in conflicts that slow down the behavioral support process. In complicated situations, the avenues for resources or administrative support may be slowed considerably. It is important to avoid implementing a behavioral support plan until critical decisions regarding training, time, tools, and opportunities for meeting are in place. Unfortunately many cases call for a swift design and implementation process.

Taking time to conduct a systems-level assessment with the functional assessment or during the design of a support plan may enhance the dialogue and problem-solving process. Time becomes an important issue when an implementation team is supporting an individual who is engaging in serious problem behavior. To work quickly and effectively, all implementation team members need to be aware of systems-level issues that create obstacles during behavior support plan implementation. Gathering information about implementation team strengths and characteristics will increase problem-solving and decision-making processes during support plan implementation. Systems-level assessment also provides information needed to create a supportive atmosphere within the implementation team by identifying important management and resource-related issues.

Assessing the Team to Promote Collaboration

Positive behavioral support involves redesigning the environment and teaching new skills; behavioral support plans can be described as a set of guidelines and directions for individuals who will implement the plan (Albin et al., 1996). Fostering a collaborative team process in positive behavioral support traditionally has not received much attention (Courtnage & Smith-Davis, 1987). The ability to work together effectively in interdisciplinary teams, however, is considered a crucial skill (Reichle et al., 1996). An implementation team's self-awareness of its strengths and needs related to positive behavioral support can promote dialogue and problem solving during the design and implementation process. Team self-assessment can consider three important variables: (a) the skill level and experience of the individuals involved, (b) the values and beliefs held by family and support providers, and (c) the stressors that affect each team member.

Skill Level and Experience of Team Members

Assessing the skills and behavior management approaches used by the individual's parents and support staff provides information important to building a plan of support. For example, some members of the team may be very confident and vocal about their ability to implement a behavioral support plan. This may overshadow the reality that other staff members providing daily support do not have the experience necessary to implement certain interventions effectively. In some cases the observations and interviews conducted during a functional assessment can identify training needed to assure a plan's success. For instance, during a functional assessment interview, a parent or other team member may request that someone with experience model how to work effectively with the individual engaging in serious problem behavior.

An implementation team member (e.g., a residential home manager or teacher) may identify specific situations where the staff under their supervision need to "unlearn" old techniques that conflict with the plan's goals (Gersten & Brengleman, 1996). The approaches currently used to manage behavioral problems may reinforce inappropriate behavior. Consider a case where an individual's problem behavior is clearly maintained by attention from staff. The implementation team is updating the functional assessment or is already gathering data indicating the problem behavior is maintained by attention. Observations and interviews may indicate that some team members have a conceptual understanding of how a problem behavior is maintained by attention, but they are not aware of how their actions directly reinforce problem behavior. An important part of the team process is recognizing and learning from the skills that each member brings to the implementation team. Effective implementation teams create an atmosphere that encourages learning and sharing of information. In this type of atmosphere, a community of learners can create a supportive situation for the change process to occur (Little, 1993). Finally, the implementation team may begin to identify key individuals who are more successful and confident than others working with problem behavior or who take the lead role in a particular setting.

Values and Beliefs Held by Family and Providers

Another assessment area involves the implementation team's awareness of the values and beliefs held by each of the individuals within the social network. Assessing the deeply ingrained assumptions or generalizations that influence the implementation team's behavior can hinder or enhance a behavioral support plan

(Senge, 1990). A behavioral support plan that is incompatible with the values and beliefs held by the individuals who will implement the plan is more likely to be abandoned or ignored (Albin et al., 1996). When strategies included in the behavior support plan have already been unsuccessfully attempted, the failure may have been related to the way that the strategy was implemented. If the majority of the implementation team does not believe that the strategy is effective, this belief may well be confirmed due to inconsistent or poor implementation. On the other hand, if the team believes that the strategy could work if implemented differently, familiarity with the process may enhance implementation efforts.

The functional assessment process usually involves a review of past behavior support strategies. Interviews and record reviews may provide important insight regarding the opinions the implementation team as a whole has about strategies attempted in the past. An implementation team member may use this information to stimulate a discussion that will lead to consensus regarding the design of the current behavioral support plan.

The values and beliefs an individual or several staff members have about their jobs can impact the success of a behavioral support plan. During the systems-level assessment, it may become clear that some individuals believe their role is that of a caretaker, whereas others see their primary function as encouraging independence. Depending upon which role is preferred, an intervention that increases an individual's opportunity for choice making and independence, for instance, may or may not be successful. Sometimes early assessment of the values and beliefs held by each member of the implementation team can help avoid conflict during the design or implementation process of the behavioral support plan. For example, the director of an agency may be confident that needed services can be provided to support an individual engaging in serious problem behavior; that is, that an alternative placement is not necessary. The other members of the social network may feel that they do not have the resources or skill necessary to support the individual but remain silent, because they do not want to disagree with their leader. This deeply held assumption, however, could result in subtle messages and behaviors that undermine progress.

Cultural differences may also lead to conflict in some situations. For instance, the values inherent in self-determination may not be embraced in other cultures where value is placed on the family as a whole and decisions are made by the head of the household. The implementation team needs to be sensitive to these differences to avoid confusion and prevent possible conflicts (Turnbull & Turnbull, 1997).

A systems-level assessment may indicate that the implementation team believes that training in specific techniques is needed. In other cases a systems-level assessment may identify values and beliefs that will likely cause discordance in the team. This information could lead to a series of discussions or training sessions intended to raise the level of awareness within the implementation team about values and assumptions that affect their behavior. Teams that are capable of having dialogues about their deeply held beliefs are more likely to be open to new ways of thinking (Senge, 1990; Senge, Kleiner, Roberts, Ross, & Smith, 1994).

Stressors That Affect Team Members

A third implementation team assessment involves the stressors that each team member may experience. As a team member, a program director or case manager may be concerned about the stress level of individuals within the social network. This may lead to a group decision to further assess and explore the level of anxiety and stress experienced by everyone within the social network. The level of stress a support staff member experiences has an impact, not only on performance, but also on the staff member's perceptions and beliefs (Hatton et al., 1999). Developing a strong supportive atmosphere may involve the use of measurement methods to raise awareness of stress levels. These assessment measures could be used later as an outcome measure related to behavioral support plan implementation.

Even stressors that are not directly related to the occurrence of problem

---

TABLE 10.2
Systems-Level Assessment Guide

Implementation Team Self-Assessment

Skill Level and Experience

- Are there discrepancies between conceptual understanding and application?

- What behavioral management strategies are currently used?

- Will training be needed before implementing positive behavioral support strategies?

- Are there staff members who tend to take a lead role when working with the individual?

- Are there opportunities for staff to dialogue and reflect on future behavioral support implementation?

- Has the group ever received training on how to work effectively in teams?

Values and Beliefs

- Can you identify key values held by each member of the team?

- Are there agency-level values that may influence a positive behavioral support plan?

continued

TABLE 10.2, *continued*

- If you have identified a potential conflict, can you determine whether all of the implementation team members are aware of this issue?
- Are there any cultural differences among the various team members that should be considered?
- How does each team member view his or her role within the social network?
- Is there a need to take some time to communicate among team members about their values and beliefs before building the behavioral support plan?

Stressors
- Is an assessment needed for each team member regarding his or her personal level of stress?
- Has there been an increase in staff turnover and absenteeism?
- Are all staff members trained in crisis management techniques?
- Does the implementation team feel confident that they can handle the emergencies that arise?
- Are there any stressors that may be unrelated to the occurrence of problem behavior (health concerns, changes within the agency)?

Assessment of Management, Resources, and Staff Development

Social Network
- Do the agencies and their consumers have mutual or competing interests?
- Can you identify activities that foster positive interactions and a sense of community?

Management and Resources
- Are there changes needed in staffing patterns?
- Are there any policies or procedures that will enhance or limit the ability of staff members to implement a behavioral support plan?
- Are there any new procedures that will increase support in the social network?
- What resources are available and who is responsible for making resource-related decisions?

Staff Development
- Are there any staff development systems in place that can assist with behavioral support implementation?
- How can the training needed for one individual be written in such a way that staff throughout an agency will benefit?

behavior can have a significant impact on the individuals providing support. Resource-related issues, changes in the structure of an agency, job dissatisfaction, and health problems are all examples of stressors that may affect an implementation team (Hatton et al., 1999). These stressors may be particularly evident in recent years, given the multiple and complex reform efforts that are so common in the human service systems that serve individuals today, including education (Gartner & Lipsky, 1987; Lipsky & Gartner, 1996), mental health (Burns & Friedman, 1990; Duchnowski & Friedman, 1990), and social services (Aber, Brooks-Gunn, & Maynard, 1995: Freeman, 1996; Freeman & O'Dell, 1993). Systems-level assessment methods that identify stressors related to an agency or system may need to explore these variables further. Table 10.2 summarizes important assessment questions that can guide the team as they explore team-related issues.

Assessing Management, Resources, and Staff Development

To be efficient, behavioral support plans must affect the systems in which people work (Anderson, Albin, Mesaros, Dunlap, & Morelli-Robbins, 1993; Baker, Dean, & Sprague, 1997). Systems-level factors related to the larger environmental issues within an agency may include assessment of (a) the entire social network, (b) management and resource-related issues, and (c) staff development systems.

Social Network

Environmental variables that influence the likelihood of problem behavior are the physical characteristics of the environment, the number of people in the environment and how they interact, and curricular or training activities (Albin et al., 1996). One can better understand how these individual environmental variables influence behavior when they are observed as existing within a larger social network or system (Baker & Freeman, 1999). Observing patterns of social interaction across staff and the individuals they support may provide information overlooked when assessing data related only to one individual and the environmental determinants of his or her behavior. For instance, assessment of activity preferences of both staff and residents may systematically improve social interaction and engagement of the residents (Baker & Freeman, 1999). Assessing the social network as the unit of analysis may provide information that can be used to increase the quality of life of all individuals in an environment.

Management and Resource-Related Issues

Another systems-level assessment involves management and resources available in an agency or system. An agency's management strategies can be indirectly related to the occurrence of problem behavior. The ways in which staffing patterns are implemented and the procedures used by an agency can enhance or detract from staff performance. Consider a case where the functional assessment provides evidence that problem behavior is likely to occur during a specific time period. The program director or home manager in a residential setting may observe that during this time period constant phone calls are coming in regarding management-related issues (e.g., nurse calls in regularly to talk about medication changes or staff members call in to leave messages).

This information may become clear while conducting observations during the functional assessment process. A home manager or other member of the social network may come to the next planning meeting with an idea for a management-level intervention approach. As a result, the implementation team decides to create a policy whereby agency members know that management-related phone calls should not be placed during time periods associated with problem behavior. This policy provides support for staff working on-site, allowing them to be free to implement interventions and work together as a team during a difficult time period.

Many agencies, whether they are schools, employment systems, or residential service providers, are under significant pressures to provide services with limited available resources. This pressure can lead staff members to assume that no resources are available, and it makes it difficult to problem solve and "think outside of the box." A systems-level assessment should include careful consideration of the existing resources and how decisions are made. Sometimes there are opportunities to temporarily shift personnel from another part of an agency to support a teacher, residential, or vocational staff person during critical time periods. In other situations informal and formal sources of support may be available to implement a behavioral support plan. In the interest of time, it may be necessary to begin dialogue concerning potential resources with key members of the implementation team during the functional assessment interview process. Beginning to think about resource options as early as possible can streamline the decisions and problem-solving process during the design of the behavioral support plan.

Staff Development Systems

Finally, assessing an agency's staff development system will help to ensure smooth behavioral support plan implementation. Being aware of the agency-wide training systems that already exist for staff members may assist the team as they consider training and support needs during plan implementation period. Assessment can reveal training materials already available within an agency that can enhance the conceptual understanding of specific behavioral support strategies. In other cases new information must be documented and packaged to ensure the longevity of a behavioral support plan (Baker, Dean, & Sprague, 1997). In either case, obtaining information about staff training mechanisms before the behavioral support plan design and implementation will create a proactive atmosphere. The second part of Table 10.2 summarizes important assessment questions that guide the implementation team as they explore management and resource-related issues in designing and implementing a behavioral support plan.

In some cases the functional assessment process begins when problem behavior has escalated to a dangerous frequency and intensity level. The implementation team is often placed in a difficult position requiring an immediate response to serious problem behavior at the same time a functional assessment is being initiated. Functional assessment of larger contextual issues may relate to an individual in crisis.

Implementing Functional Assessment and Systems-Level Assessment During a Crisis

The previous sections detailed the basic goals and various means for conducting a functional assessment. Ideally, a functional assessment is conducted before an individual's problem behaviors escalate to a point where health and safety of the individual or those within the social network are threatened. Unfortunately, this is not always possible. The methods used to conduct a functional assessment should be carefully considered when problem behavior escalates to dangerous levels.

As noted earlier, there are multiple methods available for completing a functional assessment. During a time of crisis, the time taken to implement a functional assessment can be an important consideration. Implementing a combination of indirect assessment methods, direct observations, and a functional analysis contributes to a strong functional assessment. Interviews are often the easiest functional assessment method to implement, and a variety of interview formats are available (e.g., O'Neill et al., 1997). Observations are very useful but can require some time to establish clear behavioral patterns. When behaviors are very complex and a functional pattern cannot be obtained, functional analysis manipulations may be necessary to gather more information. However, if problem behaviors have escalated to dangerously high levels, a functional analysis may not be appropriate due to the risk of serious injury.

As an added complexity, the individual in crisis may be in a temporary setting such as an inpatient psychiatric unit or a crisis respite home. This change in environment can alter the topography or function of an individual's problem behavior. When an individual has been moved to a more restrictive setting during a crisis situation, information will be needed to develop a clear transition plan outlining the resources and steps necessary to ensure a systematic and predictable return to the individual's home and community. Systems-level assessment issues are crucial during transition planning to address transitional needs and positive behavioral support planning. Planning a transition often can be facilitated by an implementation team member interviewing key staff about transportation issues, necessary schedule processes, or temporary resources. Gathering systems-level assessment information before sitting down to design the transition plan also may create a sense of predictability for the implementation team during a stressful time period.

The perceptions of the individuals within the social network and the capacity of the service setting are important variables to assess when an individual is engaging in severe problem behavior. The perception of the situation itself can vary among team members. Even the word *crisis* can have different meanings to different individuals. A crisis may mean that an individual is engaging in a problem behavior that is resulting in a constant threat to the health and safety of self or those around him or her. In another situation, a crisis may mean that there is a threat to an individual's safety during clearly defined times, followed by periods of calm. Sometimes a crisis may be agency centered rather than person centered. For example, an agency-centered crisis may occur when an individual experiences insomnia due to a medication change and lives in a residential home with staff paid to sleep through the night. The pressure placed on the agency to find staff willing to stay awake throughout the night can result in an agency-centered crisis.

A systems-level assessment can explore how the values of support staff or an entire agency can be related to problem behavior. Identification of these values can be critical, especially when rapid action is needed. An unwillingness to make changes or accommodations for a person may lead to a crisis for service providers. An agency or social network that does not place a priority on fostering an individual's opportunities for participating in community activities, building friendships, or encouraging family involvement may be creating an environment that increases the likelihood of problem behaviors.

Information regarding the values inherent in an individual's social network can be deduced through interviews with staff, observations across settings, review of records and related documents, and by implementing quality-of-life assessments. The implementation team may decide to assess the current services available, to clearly identify the resources and supports needed to stabilize a crisis. Identification of temporary resources necessary to provide support during the crisis period might include respite services or additional staff.

The information gathered will be very important to governmental employees in the educational hierarchy, social service departments, or divisions responding to the crisis. In addition, state human service personnel, case managers, school district superintendents, or service planners may be an important part of the problem-solving process as it relates to resources and administrative support. It is important to work collaboratively across these different systems to ensure consistent support and communication. It may be useful to ask the individuals at various system levels what type of information they need early in the behavioral support process. The systems-level assessment can be a means for recognizing the interdependent nature of the service systems supporting an individual in crisis while enhancing communication across service systems.

Summary

Both functional assessment and systems-level assessment are meant to enhance behavioral support plan development and implementation. Information collected during the functional assessment process must clearly identify the variables that predict and maintain problem behavior. The next step in the behavioral support plan process is to complete a competing behavior analysis and to design a plan of support. Including systems-level assessment in the design and implementation process enhances a behavioral support plan's contextual fit. Failure to assess the larger contextual variables within a system may seriously limit the effectiveness, efficiency, and longevity of a behavioral support plan. Some information regarding systems-level issues may be available naturally before the implementation team sits down to design a plan of support. Enhancing the awareness of systemic variables throughout the positive behavioral support process may increase the ease and efficiency of implementation.

Although the information needed to assess systems-level variables may appear to add work to the behavioral support planning process, many of the elements discussed can be addressed as a natural part of the design process or can be included during the implementation of indirect and direct functional assessment methods. Table 10.2 summarizes the types of questions that guide the implementation team and contribute to a systems-level assessment. Assessing systems-level issues requires the implementation team to become aware of the larger social, environmental, and systemic variables that affect behavioral support implementation.

Questions related to systems-level assessment can be incorporated into interviews or conducted during the planning process. Increased awareness during functional assessment observations may aid in the identification of important variables that enhance dialogue during the design of support. Discussions among the implementation team regarding the values, beliefs, and goals can enhance team collaboration and problem solving.

A strong emphasis inherent in positive behavioral support is designing environments that prevent problem behavior. By taking into account larger systems-related issues, the positive behavioral support process can serve as a vehicle for evaluating and improving the services available, not only for the individual engaging in problem behavior, but also for all individuals within an agency. A systems-level assessment can provide information needed to improve communication within an organization, systematically build a strong staff development system, increase an agency's ability to use outside expertise efficiently, and facilitate cross-system (i.e., multiagency) planning for resource allocation.

For instance, an agency may use the systems-level assessment process as a method for identifying what type of positive behavioral support training would benefit all staff members. An agency that hires external consultants to provide support in the behavioral support process should request that training packages be produced that can be used to train new staff (Baker, Dean, & Sprague, 1997). In some cases training information can be produced in a way that benefits all of the staff members within an organization.

Incorporating systems-level assessment strategies into an overall quality-improvement approach for an agency may enhance its ability to support individuals with serious problem behavior and create a more proactive environment for all of the individuals in the agency. By viewing the positive behavioral support process as an evaluative tool and embedding positive behavioral support assistance and training into an overall staff development approach, the implementation team will build a stronger and more proactive approach for all of the individuals they support.

References

Aber, J. L., Brooks-Gunn, J., & Maynard, R. A. (1995). Effects of welfare reform on teenage parents and their children. In R. E. Behrman (Ed.), *The Future of Children, 5*(2), 53–71.

Albin, R. W., Lucyshyn, J. M., Horner, R. H., & Flannery, B. (1996). Contextual fit for behavioral support plans. In L. Kern-Koegel, R. L. Koegel, & G. Dunlap (Eds.), *Positive behavioral support: Including people with difficult behavior in the community* (pp. 81–98). Baltimore: Paul H. Brookes.

Anderson, J. L., Albin, R. W., Mesaros, R. A., Dunlap, G., & Morelli-Robbins, M. (1993). Issues in providing training to achieve comprehensive behavioral support. In J. Reichle & D. P. Wacker (Eds.), *Communicative alternatives to challenging behavior* (pp. 363–406). Baltimore: Paul H. Brookes.

Baker, D. J., Dean, J., & Sprague, J. R. (1997). Continuous quality improvement applications in behavioral consultation. *The Behavior Therapist, 20*(7), 121–125.

Baker, D. J., & Freeman, R. L. (1999). *Staff-resident interaction patterns in community homes for persons with disabilities.* Manuscript submitted for publication.

Bijou, S., Peterson, R. F., & Ault, M. H. (1968). A method to integrate description and experimental field studies at the level of data and empirical concepts. *Journal of Applied Behavior Analysis, 1,* 175–191.

Brown, F. (1991). Creative daily scheduling: A non-intrusive approach to challenging behavior in community residences. *Journal of The Association for Persons With Severe Handicaps, 16,* 75–84.

Burns, B. J., & Friedman, R. M. (1990). Examining the research base of child mental health services and policy. *The Journal of Mental Health Administration, 17*(1), 87–98.

Carr, E. G., Langdon, N. A., & Yarbrough, S. C. (1994). Taking serious problem behaviors seriously. *Network, 4*(2), 5–14.

Carr, E. G., Langdon, N. A., & Yarbrough, S. C. (1999). Hypothesis-based intervention for severe problem behavior. In A. C. Repp & R. H. Horner (Eds.), *Functional analysis of problem behavior: From effective assessment to effective support.* Belmont, CA: Wadsworth.

Carr, E. G., & Newsom, C. D. (1985). Demand-related tantrums: Conceptualization and treatment. *Behavior Modification, 9,* 403–426.

Carr, E. G., Reeve, C. E., & Magito-McLaughlin, D. (1996). Contextual influences on problem behavior in people with developmental disabilities. In L. K. Koegel, R. L. Koegel, & G. Dunlap (Eds.), *Positive behavioral support: Including people with difficult behavior in the community* (pp. 403–423). Baltimore: Paul H. Brookes.

Carr, E. G., & Smith, C. E. (1995). Biological setting events for self-injury. *Mental Retardation and Developmental Disabilities Research Reviews, 1,* 94–98.

Courtnage, L., & Smith-Davis, J. (1987). Interdisciplinary team training: A national survey of special education teacher training programs. *Exceptional Children, 53*(5), 451–458.

Dadson, S., & Horner, R. H. (1993). Manipulating setting events to decrease problem behaviors: A case study. *Teaching Exceptional Children, 25,* 53–55.

Derby, K. M., Wacker, D. P., Sasso, G., Northup, J., Cigrand, K., & Asmus, J. (1992). Brief functional assessment techniques to evaluate aberrant behavior in an outpatient setting: A summary of 79 cases. *Journal of Applied Behavior Analysis, 25,* 713–721.

Doss, L. S., & Reichle, J. (1989). Establishing communicative alternatives to the emission of socially motivated excess behavior: A review. *Journal of The Association for Persons With Severe Handicaps, 14,* 101–112.

Drager, K., Johnston, S., Feeley, K., Freeman, R. L., Harris, M., Roberts, E., Trailor, V., Churn, S., Hicks, A., Jackson, G., Marchel, M. A., More, L., Neilsen, S., O'Keefe, A., Olive, M., Richardson, A., Smith, R., Wolff, K., & Utke, R. (1998). Functional assessment of challenging behaviors [manuscript]. In J. Reichle, M. A. McEvoy, & C. A. Davis (Eds.), *Positive approaches to managing challenging behaviors in preschoolers.* Manuscript in preparation, University of Minnesota, Minneapolis.

Duchnowski, A. J., & Friedman, R. M. (1990). Children's mental health: Challenges for the nineties. *Children's Mental Health, 17*(1), 3–12.

Durand, V. M. (1988). The Motivation Assessment Scale. In M. Hersen & A. Bellack (Eds.), *Dictionary of behavioral assessment techniques* (pp. 309–310). Elmsford, NY: Pergamon.

Durand, V. M. (1990). *Severe behavior problems: A functional communication training approach.* New York: Guilford Press.

Durand, V. M., & Crimmins, D. B. (1988). Identifying the variables maintaining self-injurious behavior. *Journal of Autism and Developmental Disorders, 18,* 99–117.

Favell, J. E., McGimsey, J. F., & Schell, R. M. (1982). Treatment of self-injury by providing alternate sensory activities. *Analysis and Intervention in Developmental Disabilities, 2,* 83–104.

Foster-Johnson, L., & Dunlap, G. (1993). Using functional assessment to develop effective, individualized interventions for challenging behaviors. *Teaching Exceptional Children, 25,* 44–50.

Freeman, E. M. (1996). Welfare reforms and services for children and families: Setting a new practice, research, and policy agenda. *Social Worker, 41*(5), 521–530.

Freeman, E. M., & O'Dell, K. (1993). Helping communities redefine self-sufficiency from the person-in-environment perspective. *Journal of Intergroup Relations, 20,* 38–54.

Freeman, R. L., Britten, J., McCart, A., Smith, C., Heitzman-Powell, L., & Sailor, W. (1999). *Foundations of Positive Behavioral Support* [On-line]. Retrieved October 19, 1999 from: www.onlineacademy.org.

Functional analysis approaches to behavioral assessment and treatment. (1994). (Special Issue). *Journal of Applied Behavior Analysis, 27,* 196–413.

Gardner, W. I., Cole, C. L., Davidson, D. P., & Karan, O. C. (1986). Reducing aggression in individuals with developmental disabilities: An expanded stimulus control, assessment, and intervention model. *Education and Training of the Mentally Retarded, 21,* 3–12.

Gartner, A., & Lipsky, D. K. (1987). Beyond special education: Toward a quality system for all students. *Harvard Educational Review, 57,* 367–395.

Gersten, R., & Brengleman, S. U. (1996). The quest to translate research into classroom practice. *Remedial and Special Education, 17*(2), 67–74.

Guess, D., Helmstetter, T., Turnbull, H. R., III, & Knowlton, S. (1986). *Use of aversive procedures with persons who are disabled: An historical review and critical analysis.* Seattle, WA: The Association for Persons With Severe Handicaps.

Hatton, C., Rivers, M., Mason, H., Kiernan, C., Emerson, E., Alborz, A., & Reeves, D. (1999). Staff stressors and staff outcomes in services for adults with intellectual disabilities: The staff stressor questionnaire. *Research in Developmental Disabilities, 20*(4), 269–285.

Horner, R. D. (1980). The effects of an environmental "enrichment" program on the behaviors of institutionalized profoundly retarded children. *Journal of Applied Behavior Analysis, 13,* 493–491.

Horner, R. H. (1994). Functional assessment: Contributions and future directions. *Journal of Applied Behavior Analysis, 27*(2), 401–404.

Horner, R. H., Albin, R. W., & O'Neill, R. E. (1991). Supporting students with severe intellectual disabilities and severe challenging behaviors. In G. Stoner, M. R. Shinn, & H. M. Walker (Eds.), *Interventions for achievement and behavior problems* (pp. 269–287). Washington, DC: National Association of School Psychologists.

Horner, R. H., & Carr, E. G. (1997). Behavioral support for students with severe disabilities: Functional assessment and comprehensive intervention. *Journal of Special Education, 31,* 84–104.

Horner, R. H., O'Neill, R. E., & Flannery, K. B. (1993). Building effective behavior support plans from functional assessment information. In M. Snell (Ed.), *Instruction of persons with severe handicaps* (4th ed.; pp. 184–214). Columbus, OH: Merrill.

Horner, R. H., Sprague, J. R., & Flannery, K. B. (1993). Building functional curricula for students with severe intellectual disabilities and severe problem behaviors. In R. Van Houten & S. Axelrod (Eds.), *Behavioral Analysis and Treatment* (pp. 47–71). New York: Plenum.

Horner, R. H., Vaughn, B. J., Day, H. M., & Ard, W. R. (1996). The relationship between setting events and problem behavior: Expanding our understanding of behavioral support. In L. K. Koegel, R. L. Koegel, & G. Dunlap (Eds.), *Positive behavioral support: Including people with difficult behavior in the community* (pp. 381–402). Baltimore: Paul H. Brookes.

Iwata, B. A., Dorsey, M. F., Slifer, K. J., Bauman, K. E., & Richman, G. S. (1994). Toward a functional analysis of self-injury. *Journal of Applied Behavior Analysis, 27*(2), 197–209.

Iwata, B. A., Pace, F. M., Dorsey, M. F., Zarcone, J. R., Vollmer, T. R., Smith, R. G., Rodgers, T. A., Lerman, D. C., Shore, B. A., Mazeleski, H. G., Cowdery, G. E., Kalsher, M. J., McCosh, K. C., & Willis, D. K. (1994). The functions of self-injurious behavior: An experimental-epidemiological analysis. *Journal of Applied Behavior Analysis, 27*, 215–240.

Koegel, L. K., Koegel, R. L., & Dunlap, G. (1996). *Positive behavioral support: Including people with difficult behavior in the community.* Baltimore: Paul H. Brookes.

Koegel, R. L., & Koegel, L. K. (1989). Community-referenced research on self-stimulation. In C. Cipani (Ed.), *The treatment of severe behavior disorders: Behavior analysis approaches* [Monograph No. 12] (pp. 129–250). Washington, DC: American Association on Mental Retardation.

Lewis-Palmer, T., Sugai, G., & Horner, R. (1999). Including high-functioning verbal students in the functional assessment process: Agreement between multiple functional assessment strategies. Manuscript submitted for publication.

Lipsky, D. K., & Gartner, A. (1996). Inclusion, school restructuring, and the remaking of American society. *Harvard Educational Review, 66*(4), 762–796.

Little, J. W. (1993). Teachers' professional development in a climate of educational reform. *Educational Evaluation and Policy Analysis, 15*, 129–151.

Lucyshyn, J. M., & Albin, R. W. (1993). Comprehensive support to families of children with disabilities and problem behaviors: Keeping it "friendly." In G. H. S. Singer & L. E. Powers (Eds.), *Families, disability, and empowerment: Active coping skills and strategies for family intervention* (pp. 365–407). Baltimore: Paul H. Brookes.

Lucyshyn, J. M., Olson, D., & Horner, R. H. (1995). Building an ecology of support: A case study of one young woman with severe problem behaviors living in the community. *Journal of The Association for Persons With Severe Handicaps, 20*, 16–30.

McClannahan, L. E., & Krantz, P. J. (1993). On systems analysis in autism intervention programs. *Journal of Applied Behavior Analysis, 26*, 589–596.

McGee, G. (1996). Discussion. In L. K. Koegel, R. L. Koegel, & G. Dunlap (Eds.), *Positive behavioral support: Including people with difficult behavior in the community* (pp. 491–494). Baltimore: Paul H. Brookes.

Meyer, L. H., & Evans, I. M. (1989). *Nonaversive intervention for behavior problems.* Baltimore: Paul H. Brookes.

O'Neill, R. E., Horner, R. H., Albin, R. W., Sprague, J. R., Storey, K., & Newton, J. S. (1997). *Functional assessment and program development for problem behavior: A practical handbook* (2nd ed.). Pacific Grove, CA: Brooks/Cole.

Reichle, J., & Johnston, S. S. (1993). Replacing challenging behavior: The role of communication intervention. *Topics in Language Disorders, 13*(3), 61–76.

Reichle, J., McEvoy, M., Davis, C., Rogers, E., Feeley, K., Johnston, S., & Wolff, K. (1996). Coordinating preservice and in-service training of early interventionists to serve preschoolers who engage in challenging behavior. In L. K. Koegel, R. L. Koegel, & G. Dunlap (Eds.), *Positive behavioral support: Including people with difficult behavior in the community* (pp. 227–259). Baltimore: Paul H. Brookes.

Senge, P. M. (1990). *The fifth discipline.* New York: Currency, Doubleday.

Senge, P. M., Kleiner, A., Roberts, C., Ross, R. B., & Smith, B. J. (1994). *The fifth discipline fieldbook: Strategies and tools for building a learning organization.* New York: Currency, Doubleday.

Taylor, J. C., & Carr, E. G. (1992a). Severe problem behaviors related to social interaction. I: Attention seeking and social avoidance. *Behavior Modification, 16,* 305–335.

Taylor, J. C., & Carr, E. G. (1992b). Severe problem behaviors related to social interaction. II: A systems analysis. *Behavior Modification, 16,* 336–371.

Tilly, W. D., Kovaleski, J., Dunlap, G., Knoster, T. P., Bambara, L., & Kincaid, D. (1998). *Functional behavioral assessment: Policy development in light of emerging research and practice.* Alexandria, VA: National Association of State Directors of Special Education (NASDSE).

Touchette, P. E., MacDonald, R. F., & Langer, S. N. (1985). A scatter plot for identifying stimulus control of problem behavior. *Journal of Applied Behavior Analysis, 18,* 343-351.

Turnbull, A. P., & Turnbull, H. R. (1997). *Families, professionals, and exceptionality: A special partnership* (3rd ed.). Upper Saddle River, NJ: Merrill/Prentice Hall.

Turnbull, H. R., & Guess, D. (1986). A model for analyzing the moral aspects of special education and behavioral interventions. In P. R. Dokecki & R. M. Zaner (Eds.), *Ethics of dealing with persons with severe handicaps* (pp. 167–210). Baltimore: Paul H. Brookes.

CHAPTER 11

Responding to Behavioral Crises by Supporting People in the Lives That They Want

Michael W. Smull
Support Development Associates
Annapolis, Maryland

People with disabilities who are frequently in crisis are often given "severe reputations" by the system that is supposed to support them. They are trapped by ways of listening and understanding that are too narrow; ways of listening that hear a need for control rather than complaints about their services. When those who receive services are not helped in getting what is important to them even as health and safety issues are addressed, when what people are asking for is mismatched with the response of the system, too often the result is people being in chronic crisis. They are trapped in a cycle where escalating behavioral complaints about services are met by escalating restrictiveness in the services provided. They are also trapped by the portrayal of their past, trapped by records that describe what did not work while recommending more of the same. The system creates a reputation that obscures the person. This chapter describes some of what my colleagues and I have learned about supporting people who have challenging behaviors and what this tells us about the need for changes in the system.

Learning From People Labeled "Not Ready" for the Community

In the late 1980s, at the University of Maryland, Susan Burke-Harrison and I were asked to help some people return to their home communities from institutions and residential schools. All of the people we were asked to help had been labeled as "not ready" for life in the community, and their records were filled with information that supported this impression. Numerous and escalating interventions had not been effective. For many there was a cycle of placement and failure. With this as their documented history, current referrals for community services had resulted in a "thanks but no thanks" response.

The records of these individuals showed years of chronic crisis and evaluation after evaluation. At first glance it would appear that the efforts to understand these individuals had been exhaustive. However, a closer look showed that there were one, two, or three kinds of evaluations being done over and over again. We listen and understand through conceptual frameworks (Brown, 1997) and the same sets of frameworks were being used over and over again. Different people were doing the evaluations, but they were not bringing different perspectives. Most of the evaluations were focused on how to make the person follow the rules of a setting that was not working. Although all of the evaluations assessed issues of health and safety, none of them explored how they might be addressed in the context of what was important to the person. Where some of what was important to the person had been learned and put in a "preferences" list, that information was then used to make the person earn what was important to them. Where people had moved to the community and had "failed" due to a lack of responsive supports, the failure was ascribed to the person rather than the system.

Those being asked to serve these individuals were sent copies of these evaluations and summaries of the efforts made to act on the recommendations within the evaluations. The inch or more of paper detailed all the reasons why the person would be challenging to serve and none of the reasons why you might like to have this person in your life. This process of "referral by packet" was done by those responsible for "placement." A broad mailing of this damning information resulted, at best, in someone willing to do more of what had not worked at a higher cost. We had inadvertently "blamed the victim," trapped people in their past, and given them reputations that reflected system deficits. We did not see that these were people who needed to be listened to differently, who needed flexible supports, and who did not fit in our existing programs.

As we spent time with these individuals we found that another way of listening to who these individuals were and what had happened told a different story. We realized that they were telling us what was important to them but were not being listened to, and they were complaining about it with their behavior. For many of these individuals, there was an unfortunate cycle that began when their complaining behavior was "targeted" and the intervention resulted in a louder complaint, followed by a more intensive interventions, and then a still louder complaint. As this cycle progressed, people were living more and more restrictive lives and shouting with their behavior. In many ways listening to them through this different framework not only taught you how these individuals needed to be supported but what was wrong with the system. As we worked with more and more people in the late 1980s and earlier 1990s, we found that (a) the behaviors that were seen as the barriers to life in the community were often nonverbal critiques of the services that they were receiving; (b) the behaviors had created a reputation, a perception; (c) and the reputation is what people saw rather than the person.

When we listened to their words and behavior, when we found and listened to those who knew them and cared about them, we discovered their desired lifestyle. We found that (a) we could learn what was important to them in how they wanted to live; (b) what they wanted was simple, doable, affordable, and different from what was typically offered to them; (c) disabilities issues that needed to be addressed could be accounted for within the context of helping people move toward their desired lifestyles.

When all of these things were done, the people with whom we were working were successful in staying in their communities and able to live lives that were more fulfilling to them (and almost always at less cost than the services that they had been receiving) (Smull & Harrison, 1992).

Learning From Colleen

Much of our early learning is captured by Colleen's story. Colleen recently received an award as self-advocate of the year. The award was given by the state official who a decade earlier had described Colleen as "too dangerous to live in the community." The Colleen of today is known for her willingness to help others, her continuously housing a series of homeless cats, and her fiercely independent spirit. When the state official first heard of Colleen, Colleen had just moved from the women's penitentiary to an inpatient unit run jointly by those of us at the University of Maryland and the state.

The view of the state official was typical of people who heard Colleen's history. No one was willing to consider Colleen for community services, because people continuously met her reputation and not the person. They heard of the person who had been incarcerated, who had hurt people. None of them had looked at how that had happened, and none of them had spent time with Colleen. When you spent time with Colleen, you met someone who would do anything for you if asked and nothing if ordered. Everyone who had spent time with her found that supporting her was not a behavioral challenge if you followed a few simple rules. Paramount among them was that no one gets in her face and tells her what to do. The second was that Colleen needed a lot of support but she needed it on her terms. When you reread her history through this lens of understanding, what had happened to her became a story of the system failing her and her reaction to that failure.

The first challenge was getting someone to meet Colleen and not just her reputation. In our early efforts, we relied on personal connections. We knew those who provided services and would call and tell them why they could be successful in supporting the person. The agency that agreed to meet Colleen is the agency that continues to support her. From the beginning they understood that with Colleen control must be shared. For example, Colleen can fire staff from her life (but not from the agency). Over time Colleen has gone from an isolated and feared person to a person who knows everyone in her neighborhood, who makes important contributions to her community.

What we accomplished was to help people learn about Colleen from a conceptual framework that was substantively different from that which they had previously been taught to use. (Some people already thought this way. For them this "new" framework gave them permission to act as they always wanted to act.) We began by asking people to not read the records before they had met the person. Instead we gave people a simple plan that introduced Colleen by describing what others liked and admired about her. It then outlined what we had learned about what was important to her. Finally, we detailed what people needed to know or do to help her get what was important to her while staying healthy and safe. What was written helped those who support her to get off to a good start. However, learning should never stop. Those who support her have learned that she must be supported to live the life that she wants, not the life that others want for her. For example, Colleen will not tolerate a traditional day program and does not want a "regular" job. Coercing her into either simply causes problems for all concerned. However, she wants to be useful and feel useful; she likes to help others. She will help a neighbor carry groceries, volunteer to work with people with complex medical needs, and interview other people who use services to see how satisfied with those services they are. Those who support her have also learned that she has to pick who will support her (and she has excellent judgment about who should be paid to work with her). Ironically the greatest current challenge in supporting someone who was once seen as dangerous is making sure that recently rescued cats move out to new homes at roughly the same rate as newly rescued cats move in.

The Order in Which Questions Are Answered Matters

One of the basic lessons that Colleen (and many others) taught us is that the questions that are asked and the order in which they are answered makes a huge difference in the outcome. In the old conceptual framework, the first question asked is how to help the person be safe and healthy. Perhaps, given the abysmal conditions in which people with disabilities were congregated when this framework was developed, it made sense to deal with issues of health and safety first. However, treating issues of health and safety as if they have no context leads to legitimizing having control over the people receiving services. Those people receiving services, who demanded that we listen to what is important to them, were also demanding that control be shared. This is emphasized in the training that we do. We tell those receiving the training that issues of health and safety must be addressed but in the context of also helping the person get what is important to him or her. We say: "Dead and happy are incompatible but alive and miserable is unacceptable." Table 11.1 contrasts the old medical-behavioral model for planning with an "essential lifestyle" approach:

Lifestyle as the Context of Importance

In the "new" way that we are looking at people, we are not ignoring issues of health and safety; we are simply recognizing that these issues always have a context. All of us address issues of health and safety for ourselves within the context of what is important to us in our own lives. Nearly all of us recognize the importance of diet and exercise and only a relative minority actually behave in a manner consistent with its importance. We then hear the rationale that because we can "make" people healthier, we should. Yet few of us would surrender control to someone else to "make" us healthier. These are complex issues. We should encourage and support, not coerce. But simply standing by when people hurt themselves or others is also unacceptable. The challenge and the ongoing struggle is how to share control and how to help those who use services have as much positive control as is possible.

We are dealing with general principles of human behavior. For people with and without disability labels, we are less likely to complain about our lives with our behavior when we have what is important to us in everyday life. In many instances identifying and addressing simple things that are important to individuals causes some health or safety issues to just go away. Where people have not been listened to for years, the solutions may be embarrassingly simple given the number of assessments and the intensity of the interventions.

One woman in the Midwest (who does not use words to communicate) was always taking her clothes off in places and in circumstances that were "problematic," including when she was outside in the winter. When those who support her listened to what was important to her, they discovered that she hates clothes that are "tight"; she wants clothes that are loose. Once she had clothes that she liked, she kept them on. As people learn to listen, they also get better and better in figuring out what people are saying.

One man (who also does not use words to communicate) will periodically yell and pound on the tray attached to his wheelchair. One of the people supporting him noticed that while he was yelling, he was also staring. She picked up the pea on the floor that he was staring at, and the yelling stopped. It seems that he feels

TABLE 11.1
Two Frameworks for Analyzing Individual Needs, Wants, and Expectations

"Old" Medical-Behavioral Framework	Alternative "Essential Lifestyle" Framework
Start with what is wrong with the person. Assess issues of health and safety. Determine what the person can and cannot do. Assess adaptive behavior; strengths and needs list. Plan how to keep the person healthy and safe; plan how to "make" her more independent.	Start with how the person wants to live. Learn what is important to the person in everyday life. Assess issues of health and safety. Assess what the person might want to learn to get more of what is important. Plan with the person. Develop a plan with the person that: • Describes what is important to the person. • Describes what others need to know or do to support the person. • Addresses any issues of health or safety in the context of how the person wants to live. • Offers opportunities for learning that help the person get more of what the person wants. • As the person is getting more of what is important in everyday life, look for opportunities for her to spend time in places and do things where she is welcomed by others. • As you build connections, look for opportunities to establish and nurture relationships. • Seek to discover what the person might like in the future and help the person move in that direction.

strongly that everything has a place and mess is not to be tolerated. Now every time he starts to yell, people ask him if something is out of place and look where he is staring. Together he and the person supporting him figure it out and the yelling stops. When people have more of what is important to them, they are more likely to work with us; as will be discussed later, they are more likely to work with us in addressing issues of health or safety.

In the old medical-behavioral conceptual model, after health and safety were addressed, we then looked at how to "make" the person more independent. These efforts to help people learn skills made enormous differences in what they could do. But the drive to help people become independent too often ignored the value of the learning to the person. Skill acquisition was the goal, regardless of the person's interest in acquiring the skill or its utility in helping the person get what was important to him or her.

Examples of these arbitrary, ineffective, and disrespectful goals are legion. Some people with disability labels continue to be told that they have to learn how to cook before they can live on their own even though increasing numbers of people without disability labels never turn their stoves on. I was once on a tour of a large public institution and saw a young man (who also did not use words to communicate) being made to sit at a table and do simple assembly, requiring one-to-one attention to do it. When I asked what the purpose was, I was told that it was an effort to get him to learn to "attend to task." When I asked how he was doing, I was told that he had doubled the time that he would "attend" and was up to 30 seconds. A bit later I saw the same young man staring intently out a window. I paused and watched him do this for the next 5 minutes. Finally I asked some of the people there what he was doing. I was told that he was watching the work-shift change and that he did this twice a day for 20 minutes at a time.

On another occasion in a day service, I saw someone teaching a person color recognition. I asked the person doing the teaching how long it had been a goal, and she said, "I don't know; I have only been here 5 years." Then I asked her what use it would be to him if he learned it, and she said, "I don't know, and I don't think I have to worry about it."

Too often we simply find out what people can't do and start mindlessly teaching, ignoring the context for the person. When I ask why they are creating goals that clearly make no sense to the person receiving services or the person providing the services, I am told that someone beyond the agency is making them do this. Although there may be pressure from those who come and inspect to have a certain number of goals across a certain number of "domains," the effects of giving in to that pressure are corrosive. If those who receive services do not like "stupid goals," they are often the recipients of programs that coerce them into compliance. Those who deliver the services learn not to question and what they learn they keep to themselves.

Learning From Jon

Jon's story illustrates how listening differently and answering these questions in a different order can make an enormous difference. Jon is an articulate self-advocate who is quite clear about what is important to him. He wants to live by himself and must have his own rituals and routines. Because he has Prader-Willi syndrome, he was placed in group homes with other people who had the same syndrome. But because what was happening in those homes was not supportive of what was important to him, he would complain with his behavior and be "asked" to leave (Bolton & Smull, 1997). Jon was among those whom Herb Lovett referred to as a "steadfast social critic" (Lovett, 1996). He had become one of the people to whom service coordinators refer when they say that 20% of the people take 80% of their time.

But what is important to Jon is modest. For example, whenever Jon gets home from work or church, he wants to change into his sweats and tennis shoes. One time when he got home from church and wanted to change, staff from the group home told him that he had to eat, because it was time for lunch. Jon did not want to get his clothes dirty and went upstairs to change anyway. When he got downstairs, he was told it was now too late for lunch. Jon got mad and told the staff with his behavior how mad he was. And Jon needed another place to live.

The people who were then asked if they could support Jon listened to him and worked with him to get an apartment where he could live with a roommate (who was subsidized). This was Jon's apartment, and he could change his clothes every time he came home, and he could eat the meals that he planned when he wanted to eat them. With Jon's agreement, his cupboards and refrigerator were locked, but he knew that he could count on people to unlock them for his planned meals. His money is in a locked box that he keeps, but he does not know where the key is kept so he cannot spend his money on food. If you ask Jon why his food and money are locked, he will tell you that they need to be, that "I don't have enough control."

The plan that was done with Jon covered this and much more. Its 15 pages describe what is important to him and what others need to know and do to support him. It tells the reader not only how to help Jon have what is important to him but how to help him maintain his weight. It notes that Jon listens to experts and that he sees his nutritionist as an expert. And it is Jon's plan; he has gone over every line. But it is not the *plan* that makes Jon's life work, it is the commitment of those who work with him to follow the plan, and it is the trust between Jon and the people who support him. As Jon said to one of the people who support him,

> "You will never leave me or take my apartment away from me. You always come back the next day when I am in a bad mood. You never threaten to stop helping me or make me move. You don't think that I am a bad or crazy person. When I am in a bad mood or having a bad day, you don't threaten to stop helping me and make me move. You don't send people away to the state hospital. You think I can live on my own. You think I can do it."

Jon's life works because the people who support Jon have continued to listen to his words and his behavior. After Jon first moved into his new apartment, he lost weight. After living there for more than a year, he began to gain weight. In talking with him, it became clear that he and his roommate were no longer getting along. Jon now lives by himself with significant drop-in support and has lost most of the weight that he gained.

Using Multiple Frameworks

For some people, discovering what is important to them is difficult, and addressing issues of health and safety within that context is extraordinarily difficult. Helping these people get lives where (a) what is important to them is present and (b) issues of health and safety are addressed takes time, commitment, and collaboration. It begins with actually doing what we often say we do but rarely carry out. We have to begin with listening and understanding. We record what we have learned and describe what we are going to do about what we learned (a simple definition of a plan). We then have to act on the plan and see how it works. As we learn from this and continue to listen, we change the plan. This person-centered learning wheel (see Figure 11.1) is what most people say they do, but most people use only a single frame of understanding (often the old medical-behavioral frame) and most are not really listening to what those who provide the day-to-day supports are learning. It appears that this is a simple process to describe but difficult to implement.

The first difficulty is in listening and understanding. There are many ways to understand someone but some are more useful for a given individual than others. Each way of understanding works better in some situations and not as well in others. Each way of understanding can be seen as a frame. As Bolman and Deale

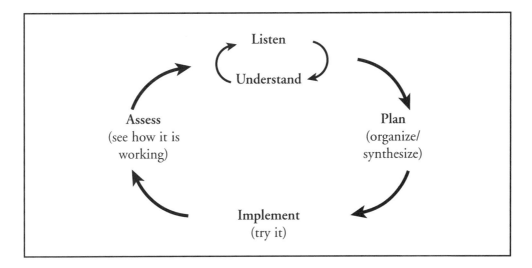

Figure 11.1. Person-centered learning wheel.

(1991) note: "Frames are both windows on the world and lenses to bring the world into focus. Frames filter out some things while allowing others to pass through easily. Frames help order our experience and decide what action to take. . . . Frames are also tools for action, and every tool has its strengths and limitations" (p. 11).

The process of using multiple frameworks is to try them, individually and in combination, to see which produce an understanding that gives the clearest picture of where you are and suggests actions that will help the person move to a more desirable future. An analogy for those of us who wear glasses is the visit to the optometrist who puts in, removes, and reverses lenses, all the while asking: "Is this better, or is this better?" Extending the analogy, the basic "lens" or overarching framework that we developed is referred to as "essential lifestyle planning."

Essential Lifestyle Planning

Essential lifestyle planning arose out of the efforts described at the beginning of this chapter. It is a structured approach to learning how someone wants to live while addressing any issues of health or safety. Each plan should be rooted in a process of learning and then communicating:

- who and what is important to the person (a) in relationships with others and their interactions, (b) in things to do and have, (c) in rhythm and pace of life, and (d) in positive rituals and routines;

- what others need to know or do (a) in helping the person get what is important to him- or herself and (b) in having a life where issues of health or safety are addressed within the context of how the person wants to live.

What is important to the person is roughly prioritized under simple headings, such as "most important" and "second in importance," and the entire plan is written everyday language so that those whose plan it is and those who implement the plan will find it easy to understand.

In training people to develop essential lifestyle plans, it is emphasized that there are four stages to the process. The first of these is called "think before you plan." Those who are going to plan are asked to answer questions that will help with understanding the purpose of the plan: what the plan is to help in accomplishing and who needs to contribute for it to be successful.

The second stage is gathering information. If the plan is to meet its purpose, you need to know what information you need to gather. If you are to discover what is important to a person, you need to have ways of gathering the information that are structured enough to guide the process and open enough to allow for the discovery of the unexpected. You also need to learn not only whom to talk with but whom to listen to.

The third stage is distilling and organizing the information gathered so that you have a plan that communicates powerfully.

The fourth stage is using the plan to move toward a desired future while continuing to learn.

Anyone whom others have significant control over where and how he or she lives has a critical need for a "living" plan, for continuous learning. The fourth stage, where the plan is used and ongoing learning is recorded, is the place where multiple frameworks can be tested. For most people, but especially those who are the subject of this chapter, overall plans are developed and then filed. They are reviewed quarterly and updated annually and rarely used in between. Many change very little from year to year. They are "dead" plans that have very little influence over how someone lives. In these instances the learning wheel shown in Figure 11.1 has broken down. In conversations with scores of people providing the day-to-day supports, I have learned that intervention plans that do not work are not implemented as they are written. Where one person is supporting several people and where the data to be collected has a high frequency, it is "estimated." Plans are reviewed and revised that are not being implemented as written and where the information on the efficacy of the intervention is not valid. Direct support staff members do tell each other what works and help each other learn. They have their own separate learning wheels. Unfortunately the only questions that those who develop and revise the plans ask of the direct support staff are questions with built-in answers, such as "Are you implementing the plan the way it was written?" "Are you taking data as you were trained?" Questions about what is really happening are rarely asked and honest answers require an atmosphere of respect and trust that is rarely present. While changes in the "target" behavior are noted, learning about what is important to the person is lost.

Real continuous learning requires that learning be seen as important and that the structures for collecting information support it. Where broad learning about someone's life takes place, the "targeted" interventions have a context and can be evaluated within that context. The basic essential lifestyle plan becomes a framework for learning. Other ways of understanding the person can be added to see what will work and how well it will work. You can address complex issues of health and safety by beginning with a frame that looks at what is important to the person and then consider different ways of understanding the issues of health and safety in the context of what is important to the person.

Harry and Complex Issues of Health and Safety

This interactive approach is illustrated by Harry's story. Harry was famous for being restrained more often than anyone in his region. He had an elaborate point-based program where he had to earn everything. When he was referred to an agency with which I was working, the core of my first suggestion was that he should just have most of what was important to him rather than having to earn it. (He had become very attached to contracts and points and those supporting him decided that having contracts and points was part of what was important to him. Therefore the scope and significance were narrowed but they were not eliminated.) For the first 3 months, this strategy seemed to work well. Harry rarely needed to be kept from hurting himself or others. Then the number of times that he would try to hurt others escalated rapidly, and he injured some people so severely that they required medical treatment. The understanding that we had of Harry was not working.

The agency supporting Harry felt that they and Harry needed a respite as well as a new understanding. They sent Harry to a new inpatient unit at the local university hospital where the staff would take another look at his issues. Several weeks later the university staff came back with a new understanding of Harry. They said that Harry had organic personality syndrome. Although Harry fits the diagnostic criteria for this label, the agency and I rejected it; this is a label that gives suggestions for management, but it offers no hope for positive change. Looking for something more hopeful, we went back and reread Harry's records. We "mined" the records (Smull & Harrison, 1992). Upon rereading them using a framework from individual service design (O'Brien & Lovett, 1992), there appeared to be another interpretation for Harry's behavior. His history suggested that there was abuse while he was a child. As an adult he sexualizes relationships with women that aren't sexual. If you couple his autism with post-traumatic stress disorder, one way of understanding his aggression is as an unusual way of seeking to be held so that he would feel safe and become less anxious. Having an external source of control and the calming effect of deep muscle pressure was something that he might be seeking. If this was true, then we, the disability service system, had created a system where he "earned" being held by being aggressive. Our efforts to give him things that were important to him had the unintended effect of making Harry work even harder to be held.

The agency that supported Harry put together a plan that acted on this hypothesis. Among a number of proposals included in this plan was the idea that male staff would ask Harry if he would like to be held whenever he appeared to be agitated and then hold him if he said yes. After some negotiation with a clinical review committee (which at first asked, "Where is the data for 'hug therapy'?") the plan was approved. Not all aspects of the plan were effective. The rented "squeeze box" just amused Harry once, and he did not use it again. By introducing a number of new elements at the same time, determining which elements had the desired effect cannot be proven. What could be demonstrated was that the frequency and severity of aggression declined dramatically and abruptly. What staff reported was that being held was a key part of the plan.

Using multiple frameworks is much easier to suggest than to do. A major part of the challenge is the single framework of understanding provided by the training of many professionals. The best trainers and the best practitioners are able to extend (and often transcend) a narrow, single way of understanding people. But too many of those doing the day-to-day work rely on the rote application of what they were taught. It is not a matter of abandoning what was learned; it is determining how it works within the context of how that person wants to live and the understanding we have of the person. The understanding that worked with Harry included seeing him as an abuse survivor as well as someone with autism. The services and supports that he received helped him learn new ways to cope as well as feel safe. While carefully thought out and applied behavioral services formed the core of the effort, the nature and content of these efforts had shifted enormously. For example, Harry's love of points and contracts was transformed into "levels" that were a way of teaching him how to monitor his own internal level of agitation and capacity to maintain control. It was the use of multiple frames or ways of understanding that created a picture of Harry that shaped those services.

It Is About Helping People Find a Better Balance

One way to help practitioners look at this is to suggest that they ask themselves the following questions:

- Is there a good balance between how the person wants to live and staying healthy and safe? Is the person (and are those who know and care about the person) satisfied with the balance?

- Where there is dissatisfaction, where things are not working, are there other ways of interpreting or understanding the issues and behaviors?

- Do any of these alternate ways of understanding the issues suggest something positive to do, something that could result in a better balance for the person?

- If we act on these alternative ways of understanding, how will we know if they are working?

Just as learning to analyze behavior using a behavioral frame is a skill, so is learning to listen to how a person wants to live. For those who practice "positive behavioral supports," it is a clearly overlapping skill, but it is sufficiently different to warrant separate training. It is a way of listening that uses a somewhat different framework, and applying that framework requires practice. It is about listening carefully and intently. This kind of listening has been labeled active listening and it is difficult (Farson, 1996). It is what has been described as a "mindful" activity (Langer, 1989). Too often there is an assumption that if you are a professional you already know how to do this. There is an expectation that you can go to a 1-day overview training of three kinds of person-centered planning, look at a couple of sample "person-centered" plans, and go forth and effectively learn how other people want to live. My experience and that of my colleagues is that it takes a rare person to pick up this new skill without extensive structured practice. It is even more challenging to apply this skill when there is a crisis. In a crisis there is no time for reflection, for puzzling something through; in a crisis there is pressure for a quick solution. Only those already skilled can apply what they know in a crisis. Applying a half-acquired skill in a crisis setting is a recipe for distortion and disaster.

A Crisis Should Not Be an Excuse

However, it is unacceptable to use "it was a crisis" as an excuse. Most crises can be anticipated. They should not come as a surprise. With most people, there is time for careful planning, for reflection. Part of the barrier is the result of a culture of chronic crisis. The officials who make decisions about where people live are typically told of someone who needs a new place to live with little lead-time, because an agency has decided to discharge, a psychiatric hospital has someone who should not be admitted, or an aging parent has been hospitalized. In these circumstances the person needs a place to sleep that night. Looking at how someone wants to live necessarily takes a "Maslowian" back seat to having shelter. But unfortunately the temporary shelter often becomes a permanent place to live, at least until that person informs us with behavior that he or she can no longer tolerate the situation into which he or she was "placed." Those who need immediate shelter (without time for planning) are telling us what is lacking in our system; however, they are seen only as "problems" that need a quick solution. There has to be a quick solution, because the officials need to move on to the next crisis. Unfortunately in a crisis culture, there is no time for reflection, for thought about real solutions, and the cycle of having today's temporary solutions adding to tomorrow's crisis is maintained.

Those who present these "problems" fall into two broad groups: those who are already well known to the system and those who are "new" to the system. People who receive services and who are complaining with their behavior about those services are typically known to those who oversee and manage the services. They are typically not just known but well-known. When they first came to the attention of the system, they were not listened to; efforts were made to have them comply with the rules of the setting. The efforts made did not work. As the person escalated complaints about the services with the escalation of the interventions, the person was "discharged" and became a "crisis." The person was then "placed" in a new setting and a new cycle began.

Learning From Crises

The officials who are asked to make the crisis "placements" have the opportunity to break what a service coordinator in Boston called "the vicious cycle of crisis." They may have to help the person move, but they can then require that evaluations be done that begin with learning how the person wants to live and look for alternative frames of understanding. The goal should be a better balance: a balance where the person has more of what is important and issues of health or safety are effectively addressed within the context of how the person wants to live. A broader analysis of the crisis typically identifies deficits in capacity. For example, there is often a need for training in the frames of understanding that we have labeled person-centered planning. Or there is a need for mental health professionals who are able to effectively evaluate and treat people with cognitive impairments. However, the greatest problem is always the absence of services and supports responsive to the issues of the person. The best officials see the challenges of those in crisis as symptoms of system deficits. These "best" officials also see the development of new capacity as one of their core responsibilities.

For those whose crisis arises because they can no longer live with their families, an important opportunity has been lost. One way to look at a system that waits until people are in crisis before offering support away from the family home is that we wait until people have lost community before we begin to build community. The time to learn what is important to the person is while that person is living with family. Many parents are happy to develop plans with their sons and daughters and to begin to act on what is being learned while they are active and able. Parents who do not have the energy to take the lead in planning still have critical information about the person.

When we wait until the parents are disabled or deceased, we have lost the information and the opportunity for building community that could have occurred. There are ways this could occur other than the funding of a large number of new service coordinators. Among the alternative solutions is to recruit some parents who are interested in acquiring the skills needed to help other parents plan and then pay these parents to help other parents develop and implement plans. Self-advocates are another neglected resource. Increasing numbers of self-advocates are being helped to develop plans on themselves. Many of them are interested, capable, and willing to assist others in developing their own plans. Parents and self-advocates may not always have the specialized clinical knowledge needed for some people to stay healthy or safe, but they make excellent partners as they almost always know how to see things through the lens of having a better life. They will almost always push for a better balance.

If this new conceptual framework is to be broadly applied, there needs to be extensive training and support in learning how people want to live and in addressing issues of health and safety in the context of what is important to the person. But there also needs to be recognition that this is a different conceptual framework and it rests on a different set of assumptions. In the old conceptual framework an often-unstated assumption was that professionals knew what was best and should make decisions for people. When this assumption is explicitly discussed, it is rationalized with concepts such as mental age, for example, "He has a mental age of 4, of course we are going to decide what is best." In saying that we know better, we ignore the fact that everyone has preferences, regardless of cognitive capacity, and we ignore the complexity of intelligence (Gardner, 1983). In a rush to an oversimplified view of self-determination, we hear the equally perverse statement: "I was in charge yesterday, but, because we now believe in self-determination, today you are in charge." The preferences that we have today are largely based on our prior life experiences. Much of what you want depends on what you have tried; an absence of opportunities narrows preferences. For all of us, choice has boundaries and control is shared, within this "new" conceptual framework what is true for the typical person is also true for those who use disability services.

In sharing control, the goal is to help the person have as much positive control as is possible. The role of the professionals and the team is to look for the best balance between what the person wants, what others want for the person, issues of health and safety, and the use of limited public resources. This is an ever-shifting balance and one that frequently has tensions between competing interests and perceptions. It does require new skills. Some of these have been discussed; others, such as the skill of negotiation, are necessary but beyond the scope of this chapter. The experiences of those who are moving down this path also indicate that acting on these concepts and using these skills requires extensive changes in policies, practices, and organizational culture. However difficult all of these efforts may seem, they are easier to accomplish and far more rewarding than seeking compliance from people who do not like where and how they are living.

References

Bolman, L., & Deal, T. (1991). *Reframing organizations: Artistry, choice, and leadership.* San Francisco: Jossey-Bass.

Bolton, C., & Smull, M. (1997). *Standing with Jon.* [On-Line]. Available: www.allenshea.com/jon.html.

Brown, J. S. (Ed.). (1997). *Seeing differently: insights on innovation.* Boston: Harvard Business School Press.

Farson, R. (1996). *Management of the absurd: Paradoxes in leadership.* New York: Simon & Schuster.

Gardner, H. (1983). *Frames of mind: The theory of multiple intelligences.* New York: Basic Books.

Langer, E. (1989). *Mindfulness.* Reading, MA: Addison-Wesley.

Lovett, H. (1996). *Learning to listen: Positive approaches for people with difficult behavior.* Baltimore: Paul H. Brookes.

O'Brien, J., & Lovett, H. (1992). *Finding a way toward everyday lives: The contribution of person-centered planning.* Harrisburg: Pennsylvania Office of Mental Retardation.

Smull, M., & Harrison, S. (1992). *Supporting people with severe reputations in the community.* Alexandria, VA: National Association of State Developmental Disabilities Program Directors.

CHAPTER 12

Evaluation for and Use of Psychopharmacologic Treatment in Crisis Intervention for People With Mental Retardation and Mental Illness

Steven G. Zelenski
Central Wisconsin Center for the Developmentally Disabled
Madison, Wisconsin

This chapter is not meant to be an exhaustive discussion of emergency psychopharmacology but rather a guide to the assessment and integrated psychopharmacological management of psychiatric and behavioral crisis in individuals with mild to moderate mental retardation. Many of the concepts draw from the mental illness literature on noncognitively impaired individuals, from geropsychiatry, and from the literature specific to intellectually disabled individuals. A flow chart accompanies this chapter to enable the reader to quickly move through the decision tree to most efficiently help the individual in crisis.

What constitutes an emergency, often associated with violent actions, frequently depends on the juxtaposition of factors relating to the individual and to the environment, rather than being intrinsic to the individual with developmental disability. In fact, when violence occurs, it is common for the individual with the disability to be a victim rather than a perpetrator. Also, when there is violence, it can be due to the individual with a cognitive disability having to resort to violence to communicate his or her victimization. Distinguishing these situations from true mental health emergencies can be difficult.

A crisis requiring intervention can be viewed either as aggression toward oneself or aggression toward others. Individuals who are not developmentally disabled usually restrict their self-aggression to suicide attempts and less commonly to self-mutilation seen with certain psychiatric disorders. The self-aggression of individuals who are developmentally disabled can be much more complex, involving the self-aggression noted above along with self-aggression of stereotypy, self-stimulation, and dysfunctional communication attempts. In addition, medical and medical-psychiatric conditions, exaggerated avoidance responses to abusive or perceived abusive situations, and developmentally appropriate impulsiveness can all play a role in the etiology of a crisis. Consideration of these factors, when possible, will improve the likelihood of an appropriate, successful intervention with minimal side effects or hazard.

The term *psychotropic* commonly refers to the entire group of medications used to alter behavior or treat psychiatric disorders. A more precise definition follows: A psychotropic is any medication that is marketed for its influence on a psychiatric or behavioral condition *or* that meets both of the following conditions: (a) it acts at the level of the central nervous system, and (b) the intent of its use is to alter signs or symptoms of a psychiatric or disruptive behavioral condition.

Factors Influencing the Use of Psychotropic Medications

Six Reasons for Using Psychotropic Medications

There are six reasons for using a psychotropic in an individual in distress from mental illness. These are (a) to treat a clearly diagnosed primary psychiatric illness, (b) to treat secondary psychiatric symptoms associated with a primary nonpsychiatric medical illness until the primary condition is treated and the symptoms resolve or until it is clear that even with treatment the psychiatric symptoms will continue, (c) to normalize nonpsychiatric but dysfunctional and emotionally painful behavior, (d) to treat medication withdrawal or discontinuation syndromes, (e) to empirically address a severely disruptive behavior that has been resistant to other interventions, and (f) to sedate an individual to allow a medical procedure when its importance is unquestioned and the procedure cannot be performed without the sedation. In this chapter the use of medications in a, b, c, and e above will be addressed. It is important to emphasize that an abusive use of medications can occur if caregivers or even patients themselves view chronic situations in a crisis context and use crisis response as a substitute for careful evaluation and treatment.

Influence of Underlying Medical-Psychiatric Disorders on
Behavioral Genetic Disorders

Many other sources have outlined the behavioral phenotypes associated with known genetic disorders and these won't be examined in detail here. An excellent review is available in the book *Developmental Neuropsychiatry* (Harris, 1995). To illustrate the importance of awareness of predisposing factors, consider Prader-

Willi syndrome, one of the five most common syndromes seen in birth-defects clinics. Key psychiatric features of this syndrome include compulsive food-seeking, irritability, anger, a low frustration tolerance, and stubbornness. Frequently these features are a part of the basis of day-to-day functioning, but occasionally they may combine to yield a significant dysfunctional and violent episode. Knowing this can prepare caregivers for a potentially disruptive episode and allow for readiness that may ultimately minimize the need for maximally invasive and risky interventions. Unfortunately, there are few studies that suggest the best pharmacologic interventions based on genetic factors; thus the treating physician must rely on personal experience and nonspecific interventions. However, if the genetic disorder affects metabolism in some way — possibly by altering hepatic metabolism or renal excretion as may occur in tuberous sclerosis — this knowledge prepares the clinician to offer only the safest interventions in an emergency.

Developmental Disorders

The developmental age of the individual in crisis is an important consideration. At times, physicians are asked to intervene psychopharmacologically when the so-called dysfunction is not really dysfunctional if the patient's baseline developmental functioning is included in the evaluation. Unfortunately, while this may provide an explanation for the disruptive situation, many times intervention is still required because of the physical development of the individual. An example of how this consideration will lead to different interventions for similarly appearing behaviors is presented in the two following cases.

Joe is 45 years old and is developmentally disabled because of childhood physical abuse. Radiologic evaluation of his brain reveals injury to the frontal cortex and left parietal areas. This has left Joe with minimal mental retardation, but little abstracting ability and little insight for problem solving, with a developmental age estimated at about 6 years. At his worksite Joe has functioned well and is generally well liked by coworkers and supervisors. Recently a new employee was hired, one who tends to be a bully and who has been making fun of Joe. The supervisors have tried to curtail this, but the employee continues to find covert opportunity. On one such occasion, Joe reached his limit and attacked the employee, similar to a first-grader striking back at a taunting classmate. Unfortunately, Joe was fired from his job and a court investigation is under way to determine if charges will be filed. Joe has been staying at his group home most of the day and shows increased irritability. Several times he has struck out at peers and staff. The physician was consulted for recommendation of medication for crisis intervention to control his "acute" violent behavior.

Mary is 26 years old and is developmentally disabled because of Soto's syndrome. She has no evidence of any endocrine disorder, nor is there any brain radiologic evidence of abnormality. Mary can be social and pleasantly interactive, but she recently was destructive at her apartment and responded very aggressively to the police who were called by neighbors to investigate the noise. She attacked one of the investigating officers and was brought to jail, where a psychiatrist is assessing her. He cannot approach her because of the violent outbursts directed at anyone in her proximity.

In Joe's case a team evaluation revealed the presence of a major depression, and no crisis medication was introduced. Instead, a combination of cognitive therapy and an antidepressant was used, along with increased support from his case manager. In Mary's case the team recognized that aspects of brain damage of Soto's syndrome could have been a major predisposing factor leading to behavior beyond Mary's control, and a combination of oral risperidone (Risperdal) and lorazepam (Ativan) was given for her safety and to allow further evaluation.

From these cases, we begin to see the importance of multiple factors in assessing and treating acute dysfunctional behaviors in an individual with a developmental disability. Following is a further discussion of the appropriate use of psychotropic medications in complex clinical presentations.

Psychotropic Medication as Part of the Multidisciplinary Approach

Medical Disorders

In the individual with developmental disability and mental illness, a fragile balance exists between already disrupted but basal physical functioning and the dysfunction of acute illness — whether physical or psychiatric. In a brain already sensitized by prior injury, what might not be of concern in the typical brain becomes a traumatic insult. A physician should always suspect physical explanations for any acute psychiatric signs or symptoms when working with a patient with developmental disability. Table 12.1 lists some of the common physical causes of psychiatric symptoms.

TABLE 12.1

Common Physical Causes of Apparent Psychiatric Signs and Symptoms

---

HURTS:

Head

Urinary tract

Reflux and other GI factors

Thyroid

Seizures

General Medical Conditions

In evaluating whether a general medical condition is responsible for a particular behavioral or psychiatric crisis, several important clinical clues are available. These include (a) the age of the first episode not being characteristic of the apparent condition, (b) the presence of coexisting physical illness known to cause psychiatric or behavioral symptoms (see Table 12.1 for a useful acronym), (c) a poor response to multiple psychotropic interventions, (d) a lack of family history of psychiatric illness, (e) a single acute episode, or (f) a change in mental status. While none of these clearly indicates a general medical condition as causing the crisis, they provide presumptive evidence suggesting further medical evaluation. Personal experience has revealed that approximately 15% of psychiatric referrals in a general population have a general medical condition that explains the psychiatric signs or symptoms, and more than 75% of psychiatric referrals in a mildly and moderately mentally retarded population have a general medical condition that could explain or contribute to the psychiatric signs or behavioral dysfunction responsible for the referral. Many of these were previously unrecognized medical conditions, such as infection, musculoskeletal problems, thyroid, and vision or hearing loss. Hall (1980) found that 5% of psychiatric patients had unrecognized medical disorders that were causative of psychiatric symptoms; 21% of patients had concomitant medical illnesses contributing to the psychiatric symptoms; and physical disease was found causing psychiatric symptoms in 42% of psychiatric outpatients.

Seizure Disorders

Seizure-Related Behaviors — Seizure disorders have frequently been implicated in behavioral changes. The changes can be acute or chronic and can be debilitating and frequently difficult to diagnose (Manford et al., 1988). Partial seizures of the temporal or frontal lobe are most often implicated. These can resemble primary psychiatric illnesses, including psychoses, mood disorders, panic disorder, and dissociative disorders (Deonna,1995; Tisher et al., 1993).

Interictal Behaviors — Less widely recognized are the long-standing personality (Swanson, Rao, Grafmen, Salazar, & Kraft, 1995) and behavioral changes that occur between seizures, which can lead to increased irritability and lowering of frustration threshold (Gerald, Spitz, Towbin, & Shantz, 1998).

Psychiatric Disorders

Psychiatric diagnosis in a developmentally disabled individual can be complicated by both "shadowing" effects and communication and insight gaps (Giacino & Cicerone, 1998). Individuals with learning disabilities may experience subsequent head injury, further impairing their abilities (Donders & Strom, 1997). This can lead to a long history of inadequate psychiatric diagnosis improperly guiding medication decisions. In addition, little attention has been paid to the experience and ability of caregivers to help in the process of assessment. Hastings (1997) revealed that experienced care staff and inexperienced students differed in their views on likely causes of challenging behaviors. The experienced staff as a group rated social and emotional variables as likely causes of challenging behaviors, while the inexperienced group was more likely to attribute difficulties to more immediate causes.

Personal experience suggests that experienced nonmedical staff tend to view social and environmental factors as significantly involved in crisis behaviors, while inexperienced nonmedical staff expect a physician or psychiatrist to be able to "fix" a problem. Inexperienced medical staff tend to try to do what they are asked. This has profound implications for psychopharmacologic interventions in crisis situations, because the prescribing physician may be unduly influenced by inaccurate information and the urgings of inexperienced staff.

Psychotropic Medications in Empiric and Crisis Use
What is commonly called "crisis" can be further defined as Types I and II. Type I crisis is acute and dangerous to self or others. Type II crisis is disruptive and interferes with quality of life and social interaction, but it is short-lived and not necessarily dangerous. To be effective, psychopharmacologic interventions must be geared to the type of crisis as well as to the suspected etiology. Typically, Type II crises do not require acute psychopharmacologic interventions.

Rapid Assessment
In a crisis, rapid assessment must be made of a potential treatable pain etiology for the acute behavior. Common sources of pain that might lead to a Type I crisis are acute abdominal pain, cluster migraine headaches, and renal colic. Pain as an etiology for apparent acute psychiatric decompensation is more likely when the individual with a disability has communication limitations. Clearly, rapid assessment is the key, followed by an emergency room evaluation. In the case of a woman, always perform a pregnancy test, as the results may influence the types of intervention, particularly medications that may be available. Other medical conditions that could be likely causes of a Type I crisis are respiratory difficulty and cardiovascular problems. Typical causes of pain and discomfort that may lead to a Type II crisis are gastrointestinal reflux, premenstrual syndrome, hunger, tight or ill-fitting clothes, and headache.

Treatment Options
If an acute general medical crisis does not appear to be the immediate, treatable cause of the behavioral-psychiatric crisis, a combination of physical management and psychotropic medication is appropriate. If psychotropic medications are used,

several options are available. If the individual is willing and able to take oral medications, a short-acting benzodiazepine, such as lorazepam (Ativan), or a longer-acting benzodiazepine, such as diazepam (Valium), can be provided. Emergency room experience suggests that in a situation that is difficult to control, a combination of lorazepam and haloperidol (Haldol) can be even more rapidly effective (Bieniek, Ownby, Penalver, & Dominguez, 1998). Risperidone is an alternative to haloperidol when the oral route is available (Perry, Pataki, Munoz-Silva, Armenteros, & Silva, 1998; Zelenski). An alternative to the benzodiazepines are the antihistamines hydroxyzine (Vistaril) or diphenhydramine (Benadryl), although recent evidence in adolescents suggests that the only effect of these medications is a placebo effect or a "needle effect" when administered intramuscularly. The individual's past response to medications and the physician's experience and comfort with specific medications will help decide the best choices.

Prior consent may not be required in the case of a single-episode emergency use of a psychotropic medication (see local law), but the forcible administration of psychotropic medications is typically problematic. Each facility and treating physician should have legal counsel and an established procedure prior to attempting to initiate forcible administration in a crisis situation.

Specific Medications Options by Drug Class

The following is a discussion of optimum use of crisis medications in each major class of psychotropics.

Neuroleptics — Many current clinicians feel that there is minimal value in the older or "typical" antipsychotics as the first line of treatment for psychosis or severe disruptive behavior. This is based on the improved side-effect profile of newer, atypical medications and the apparent lower risk of extrapyramidal symptoms, as well as lowered long-term risk of tardive dyskinesia. When used in a crisis situation, preference is given to shorter-acting medications, such as a .5 mg to 4 mg dose of risperidone. Unfortunately, this medication does not have a parenteral formulation, and haloperidol, an older, high-potency, more typical neuroleptic, is the preferred medication when parenteral administration is necessary. The dosage can range from .5 mg to 20 mg. With both medications, side effects become more frequent as the dosage is increased.

Antiepileptics — The medications primarily on the market for seizure control have in recent years been found to be very effective in treating individuals with some mood disorders as well as those with impulse-control disorders. Naturally, if the disruptive behavior is seizure-related, these medications can be extremely valuable in treating the underlying seizure disorder as well. While several of these medications can be used parenterally as well as orally, valproic acid (Depakote) may have the greatest usefulness in aborting a crisis situation, especially one associated with a manic episode. It can be given in loading doses to attain therapeutic blood levels rapidly, and thus achieves the desired clinical effect. It is also available in a parenteral form. Two important side effects, while infrequent, must be considered. These are acute hepatic toxicity and pancreatitis — with the hepatic failure being more common. The newer antiepileptic medications, such as lamotrigine (Lamictal), may eventually prove effective in a crisis situation, but no research is currently available to support this use.

Antidepressants — Although oral antidepressants typically are not useful in acute situations, there is evidence that some may be helpful parenterally for the acute treatment of depression. Both imipramine (Tofranil) and amitriptyline (Elavil) are available parenterally for this indication. Additionally, certain antidepressants, such as trazodone (Desyrel), may be effective for the acute treatment of explosive behaviors (Zubieta & Alessi, 1992), and amitriptyline can be used as a short-term sedative when a benzodiazepine is contraindicated. These medications also have the advantage that if they are effective in a crisis situation, they may be continued chronically with some hope of effectiveness (Bernstein, 1992; Gedye, 1991; Pinner & Rich, 1988; Singh, 1993).

Anxiolytics and Sedatives — The most commonly used medications in crisis situations have typically been the benzodiazepines. These medications are relatively safe, with no long-term problems other than possible addiction. Short-term side effects usually consist of sedation, which is typically a desirable effect. The problems of respiratory depression are infrequent and can be reversed. One problem with benzodiazepines in an individual with developmental disability has been the occurrence of paradoxical excitement and disinhibition (Weisman, Berman, & Taylor, 1998). Additionally, unusually high doses can sometimes be required because of a long history of concurrently administered hepatic enzyme-inducing anti-seizure medications. Therefore, some usefulness for the sedating antihistaminic preparations, such as hydroxyzine (Vistaril) and diphenhydramine (Benadryl), has been reported. Unfortunately, the relatively safe and well-tolerated atypical anxiolytic buspirone (Buspar) appears to be of little benefit in an acute situation.

Aphaadrenergic Agonists — Clonidine (Catapres) is prescribed primarily for its antihypertensive action. However, it is also useful because of its general calming and sedating effect as well as for its potential for long-term use for attention deficit disorder, fragile X syndrome, and other hyperarousal behaviors, anxiety, aggression, and general hyperactivity.

Beta-Adrenergic Blockers — These medications (e.g., propranolol [Inderal] and atenolol [Tenormin]) have a long history of use in psychiatric disorders, initially for performance anxiety. These medications are primarily marketed for treatment of cardiovascular disorders. An important side effect is their impact on pulmonary function and, when used as a psychotropic, their effect in lowering blood pressure. Their usefulness ranges from acute treatment of anxiety disorders to psychotic disorders, impulse control disorders, aggression, and akathisia.

Precautions
Whenever emergency use of a psychotropic is initiated, certain precautions are needed. These are outlined in Table 12.2.

After the crisis, appropriate measures regarding the future should be taken. These include further evaluation into the reason for the crisis as well as the development of a plan for future crisis response.

Medication Side Effects Mimicking Disruptive Behaviors
Much like geriatric patients, individuals with developmental disabilities frequently show physiologic and pathologic changes that may make them particularly susceptible to the neuropsychiatric and medical complications of medications. When affected, the most obvious changes may be in mental status — with signs of delirium — or in a variety of behavioral changes. These problems often

---

TABLE 12.2
Precautions When Administering an Emergency Psychotropic

Administer drugs in doses appropriate to body weight.

Use lower dose in older patients.

Monitor vitals before and after administering medication.

Be aware of the seizure history of the patient.

Avoid long-acting antipsychotic medications in patients not previously exposed to them.

Avoid antipsychotics in patients with heart disease.

If benzodiazepines are used, have flumazenil available in case of respiratory depression.

If antipsychotics are used, have IV diphenhydramine available for acute dystonic reactions.

are unrecognized and are mistakenly treated with psychotropics. A rapid assessment of medication history can avoid this mistake.

Acute Drug-Induced Behaviors

The most common — but frequently unrecognized — complication of neuroleptic treatment is akathisia. This can occur with a variety of medications, including antipsychotics, antidepressants, and metoclopramide (Reglan). Frequently, the physician's response is to increase the dose of offending medication to deal with the new crisis. This usually worsens the behavior, leading to further increases in the medication. It is very important to always keep this phenomenon in mind and consider reducing the potentially offending medication while treating the disruptive behavior with an alternative medication.

Anticholinergic medications are associated with delirium more than any other drug class (Tune, Carr, Hoag, & Cooper, 1992). This usually results from the use of multiple medications, each contributing an anticholinergic effect which, used alone, may have no detrimental effects. Simplifying medication regimes and being sensitive to this potential additive effect is key to avoiding this problem.

Other potentially dangerous medications are digoxin (Lanoxin) and cimetidine (Tagament). Digoxin can easily reach toxic levels, leading to mental status changes and hallucinations. Cimetidine can lead to psychosis, particularly when used intravenously. Although certain antiseizure medications are potentially useful in treating explosive behaviors, the antiepileptic medication phenobarbital (Barbita) has long been implicated in a disinhibition syndrome in certain individuals. With the advent of newer, effective antiseizure medications, phenobarbital is being used less frequently. However, one of the newer medications, lamotrigine (Lamictal), has been implicated in provoking aggressive behavior and violence in intellectually handicapped patients with epilepsy (Beran & Gabson, 1998). Gabapentin (Neurontin) has also been implicated in causing the development of behavioral side effects, including intensification of baseline behaviors and the development of new behavioral problems, including aggression (Lee et al., 1996). Treatment of these behaviors is complicated by the inability of the treating physician abruptly to withdraw the offending medication for fear of inducing a recurrence of seizures. In this case, an antiseizure benzodiazepine (e.g., diazepam [Valium]) that will help sedate the individual during the crisis would be an appropriate course while a crossover to a less offensive antiseizure medication is achieved.

Drugs of Abuse and Over-the Counter Medications

Often neglected as potential causes of drug-induced behaviors are the drugs of abuse or combinations of over-the-counter medications with prescription medications and natural products. The most effective way to look for drugs of abuse and/or over-the-counter stimulants is with a combination of a urine and serum toxicological screen. A careful history by a trusted friend or family member can also be helpful.

Summary

Treating an individual who has a developmental disability and who also is suffering from a disruptive behavioral experience can be a complicated but key part of providing the highest quality of care possible. In a crisis, nothing seems to be what it appears, yet rapid, accurate assessment and treatment are frequently injury- or even life-sparing. Mistakes will be made but should not discourage attempts to help. A key factor in minimizing mistakes is gathering as much information and medical and biopsychosocial history as possible prior to a crisis. Once a crisis has occurred, the treatment team should conduct an extensive evaluation of the outcomes of any interventions, with an eye to developing an improved plan if further crises occur. Having experienced clinicians available for rapid assessment at the time of crisis is helpful and, in lieu of this, having team members readily available and trained in crisis intervention is critical. The goal always must be to minimize harm and maximize the benefit of intervention.

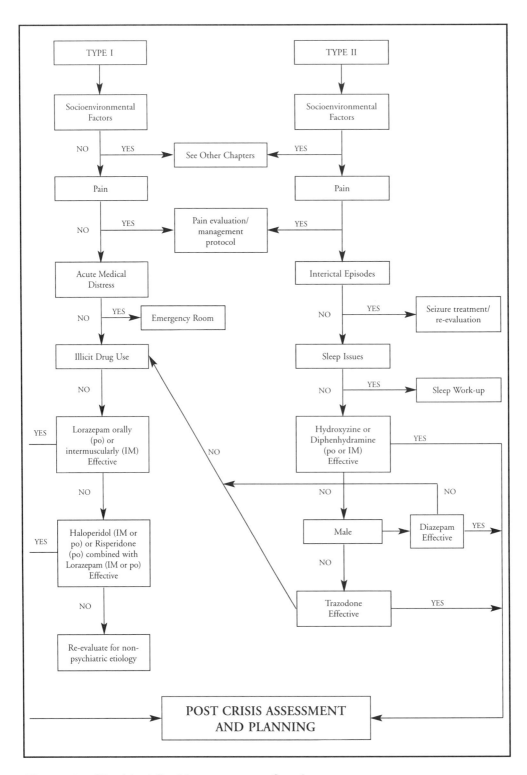

Figure 12.1. "Psychiatric" crisis management flowchart.

References

Beran, R. G., & Gibson, R. J. (1998). Aggressive behaviour in intellectually challenged patients with epilepsy treated with lamotrigine. *Epilepsia, 39,* 280–282.

Bernstein, L. (1992). Trazodone treatment of targeted aggression in a mentally retarded man. *Journal of Neuropsychiatry and Clinical Neurosciences, 4,* 348.

Bieniek, S. A., Ownby, R. L., Penalver, A., & Dominguez, R. A. (1998). A double-blind study of lorazapam versus the combination of haloperidol and lorazepam in managing agitation. *Pharmacotherapy, 18,* 57–62.

Deonna, T. (1995). Cognitive and behavioral disturbances as epileptic manifestations in children: An overview. *Seminars in Pediatric Neurology, 2,* 254–260.

Donders, J., & Strom, D. (1997). The effect of traumatic brain injury on children with learning disability. *Pediatric Rehabilitation, 1,* 179–184.

Gedye, A. (1991). Serotonergic treatment for aggression in a Down's syndrome adult showing signs of Alzheimer's disease. *Journal of Mental Deficiency Research, 35,* 247–258.

Gerard, M. E., Spitz, M. C., Towbin, J. A., & Shantz, D. (1998). Subacute postictal aggression. *Neurology, 50,* 384–388.

Giacino, J. T., & Cicerone, K. D. (1998). Varieties of deficit unawareness after brain injury. *Journal of Head Trauma Rehabilitation, 13,* 1–15.

Hall, R. C. W. (Ed.). (1980). *Psychiatric presentations of medical illness.* New York: SD Medical and ScienFic Books.

Harris, J. C. (1995). *Developmental neuropsychiatry: Assessment, diagnosis, and treatment of developmental disorders* (Vol. 2). New York: Oxford University Press.

Hastings, R. P., Reed, T. S., & Watts, M. J. (1997). Community staff causal attributions about challenging behaviors in people with intellectual disabilities. *Journal of Applied Research in Intellectual Disabilities, 10,* 238–249.

Lee, D. O., Steingard, R. J., Cesena, M., Helmers, S. L., Riviello, J. J., & Mikati, M. A. (1996). Behavioral side effects of gabapentin in children. *Epilepsia, 37,* 87–90.

Manford, M., Cvejic, H., Minde, K., Andermann, F., Taylor, L., & Savard, G. (1998). Case study: Neurological brain waves causing serious behavioral brainstorms. *Journal of the American Academy of Child and Adolescent Psychiatry, 37,* 1085–1090.

Perry, R., Pataki, C., Munoz-Silva, D. M., Armenteros, J., & Silva, R. R. (1997). Risperidone in children and adolescents with pervasive developmental disorder: Pilot trial and follow-up. *Journal of Child and Adolescent Psychopharmacology, 7,* 167–179.

Pinner, E., & Rich, C. L. (1988). Effects of trazodone on aggressive behavior in seven patients with organic mental disorders. *American Journal of Psychiatry, 145,* 1295–1296.

Singh, A. N. (1993). Case report 2: Fluoxetine treatment of self-injurious behaviour in mental retardation and its interaction with carbamazepine. *Journal of Drug Development, 6,* 23–24.

Swanson, S. J., Rao, S. M., Grafman, J., Salazar, A. M., & Kraft, J. (1995). The relationship between seizure subtype and interictal personality. Results from the Vietnam Head Injury Study. *Brain, 118*(1), 91–93.

Tisher, P. W., Holzer, J. C., Greenberg, M., Benjamin, S., Devinsky, O., & Bear, D. M. (1993). Psychiatric presentations of epilepsy. *Harvard Review of Psychiatry, 1,* 219–228.

Tune, L., Carr, S., Hoag, E., & Cooper, T. (1992). Anticholinergic effects of drugs commonly prescribed for the elderly: Potential means of assessing risk of delirium. *American Journal of Psychiatry, 149,* 1393–1394.

Weisman, A. M., Berman, M. E., & Taylor, S. P. (1998). Effects of clorazepate, diazepam, and oxazepam on a laboratory measurement of aggression in men. *International Clinical Psychopharmacology, 13,* 183–188.

Zelenski, S. G. (1999). *Risperidone in the management of acute self-abusive crisis in individuals with severe and profound mental retardation.* Unpublished manuscript.

Zubieta, J. K., & Alessi, N. E. (1992). Acute and chronic administration of trazodone in the treatment of disruptive behavior disorders in children. *Journal of Clinical Psychopharmacology, 12,* 346–351.

CHAPTER 13

Building an Effective Team for Crisis Prevention and Response

Norman A. Wieseler
Eastern Minnesota Community Support Services
Faribault, Minnesota

Ronald H. Hanson
Mount Olivet Rolling Acres
Victoria, Minnesota

The change in the last decade from the traditional manner of diagnosis of mental retardation to the newer emphasis on functional skills has highlighted the importance of the interdisciplinary team in assessment and treatment planning. Previously, the diagnosis was made by focusing on the cognitive and adaptive skill deficits occurring during the developmental period of below age 18 years (Grossman, 1983). The major shift was a change in focus to a functional model examining the interaction of a person with limited intellectual ability and the person's environment (American Psychiatric Association, 1994; Luckasson et al., 1992). This entails identifying areas of support the individual needs to succeed in community integration and prosper with an enhanced lifestyle. Ten possible adaptive areas that may require support are enumerated in the American Association on Mental Retardation guidelines (Luckasson et al., 1992): communication, self-care, home living, social skills, community use, self-direction, health and safety, functional academics, leisure, and work. Rather than making a diagnosis of mild, moderate, severe, or profound mental retardation, these newer guidelines center on the extent supportive services are necessary. These supports are categorized as intermittent, limited, extensive, and pervasive. For example, an individual with two supports needing only intermittent assistance may need help only in self-direction and functional academics. Alternatively, an individual needing pervasive supports may need assistance in all 10 areas of adaptive functioning. The greater the level of support required, the more services from a variety of professionals and caregivers are needed. Without the intervention of these services, care may be splintered, neglecting service needs or delivering inconsistent interventions across various disciplines.

This chapter describes the characteristics of an effective team for people with developmental disabilities and the manner in which collaboration is developed and maintained. It describes how a productive interdisciplinary team meeting should be conducted and how the integrated service plan can be efficacious during crisis prevention and response.

Components of an Effective Interdisciplinary Team

A behavior requiring crisis prevention and response is one "that results in self-injury or injury of others, causes damage to the physical environment, interferes with the acquisition of new skills, and/or socially isolates the learner" (Doss & Reichle, 1991, p. 215). Essential to crisis response and prevention is the development of an individual's crisis prevention plan. Each plan is individually tailored to address the procedures to be followed and who will be responsible for implementing the predetermined procedures. Challenging behaviors usually occur in a social environment. Consequently, it is important for the interdisciplinary team to isolate the environmental contextual variables and their interaction with the client's psychological and physical characteristics. Developing a crisis prevention and response plan requires the collaborative efforts of the team to avoid ineffectual management of the crisis.

Members Support One Another's Efforts

A cohesive team effort requires certain characteristics. First, members of the interdisciplinary team actively support one another's efforts; that is, each team member actively works to achieve the goals germane to his or her discipline by cooperating and supporting the other team members' efforts. For example, the psychologist values the work of the speech therapist by appreciating the therapist's effort during the meeting. This "positive interdependence" is the foundation of effective teams (Rainforth & York-Barr, 1997). It requires a shared purpose while clarifying each member's role and responsibility. Because "positive interdependence" is an evolving process in interdisciplinary teams, opportunities to work collaboratively facilitate the team's working as a unit with common goals.

Strategies for Developing a Seamless Team, Sharing Values

Another characteristic of an effective interdisciplinary team is that the members share core values. Thus a "seamless service system" becomes possible (Griffiths & Nugent, 1998); these authors describe 10 strategies to develop a seamless team with the common aim of producing individualized client-centered goals and preventing or skillfully managing future crisis situations.

The first strategy recommended by Griffiths and Nugent is the designation of a coordinator. This role is essential to the organization of the interdisciplinary team and ensures a plan for crisis prevention and response. The coordinator arranges for interdisciplinary team meetings, invites participants, chairs the meeting, and ensures ongoing communication among team members. The coordinator is often the case manager, but others may assume the role. At times, it may be helpful to have the psychologist, program director of a facility, or a parent assume the coordinator role.

The second strategy calls for the involvement of all the relevant individuals on the team. This would include family members, caregivers, and professionals (e.g., behavior analysts, nurses, physicians, psychologists) critical to the crisis prevention planning and response. To be effective team members, they must share the values of the team, and work within the context of the resources available to the client's residence and worksite. If members are unable to attend a scheduled meeting, it is important they receive meeting minutes from the interdisciplinary team to stay informed.

Obvious, but often overlooked, is the overt recognition of the contributions of all team members. This third strategy is key to seamless service delivery. Usually, valuable information is obtained from the primary caregiver who is most familiar with the client's behavior patterns. It is important that the team acknowledge that each member of the team differs in his or her experience with the client and that the various disciplines bring differing perspectives to the table. These differences in views and experiences can provide divergent and creative ideas for developing the crisis prevention and response plan.

The fourth strategy involves working together to discover the client's personal goals to improve his or her quality of life. The explicit articulation of personal goals often depends on the individual's functioning level; however, an appreciation of the client's personal goals is an essential element in the service plan development. One method of discovering the client's personal goals is through person-centered planning. In the past few years, a variety of processes have been developed, but they share many common elements. For example, most are developed with large sheets of paper and markers that record the statements of the focus client and key individuals in that person's life in both the personal profile and the personal planning sessions. All person-centered planning focuses on developing an enhanced future for the client. Kincaid (1996) has enumerated five outcomes for person-centered planning. First, the client must live in the community and participate in community life as others without intellectual disabilities. For example, the client must be able to shop, eat in a restaurant, view a movie, or visit friends. Second, the client must be supported in acquiring and maintaining relationships with others in the community. By adhering to this outcome, the client will have healthy interactions with friends and family on a recurring basis. Third, the client must be able to make choices, both on minor and major decisions, about his or her life. That is, not only will the client decide when, what, and where to eat, but other decisions will also be embraced. These include where to work, where to live and with whom, and how to spend money. At times, seemingly minor elements of daily life are major for the client. For example, a client may prefer to bathe at night rather than in the morning. When the client's personal preference for evening bathing was honored, previous tantrum episodes related to morning bathing dissipated. Although the client was unable to articulate his preference, knowing and honoring his preferences were effective in preventing challenging behavior. Violation of personal goals or preferred daily routines may make a crisis behavior more likely. Fourth, the client must be allowed the opportunity to gain dignity and respect in the community. The person will be supported in making contributions to the community that result in community recognition as a valued member of society. Fifth, the client will be supported in developing personal competencies. For example, learning new skills not only produces an attitude of achievement, it also results in enhanced self-worth. Kincaid (1996) concludes that assessment and planning are an ongoing process necessary throughout the client's life and changes whenever the client experiences a differing lifestyle.

A fifth team strategy for developing a crisis prevention and response plan is the completion of a functional assessment. A complete functional assessment examines both the environmental influences and the biomedical and psychological factors. A multimodal assessment considers the biopsychosocial influences of behavior and identifies the instigating conditions, vulnerability influences, and functional influences on behavior potentially resulting in a crisis situation (Gardner, 1998a).

The sixth team strategy is the development of a comprehensive behavioral support plan. A component of the plan focuses on personal goals, but also addresses crisis prevention and response. The support plan contains interventions of a short-term (i.e., crisis response) and long-term nature (i.e., crisis prevention). The comprehensive support plan emanates from the information contained in the assessment. All of the interdisciplinary team members endorse the components of the support plan and assist in its development. The plan must be well understood by all caregivers who interact with the client.

The seventh team strategy is the evaluation of the behavioral support plan using observable and measurable outcomes. This data-based monitoring provides useful information on the overall frequency of behaviors targeted for intervention and evaluates the effectiveness of the support plan components. If psychotropic (Kern, 1999) or anticonvulsant medications (Gates, 1999) are prescribed, these interventions are also evaluated for positive or adverse effects on behavior.

Optimal communication among all members of the interdisciplinary team is the eighth strategy. Information concerning the support plan, medication's effects, side effects, and the overall client's demeanor are types of important information for team members. The coordinator is responsible for transmitting this information to others who provide direct or professional care for the client. If the client's situation has not improved, the team members must be informed and meet to design alternatives or modify the current interventions.

The ninth strategy, regular scheduled interdisciplinary team meetings, is important to enhance communication and guarantee the commitment of all team members. These regularly scheduled meetings assure that information transfer occurs in a timely manner and any modification in the client's support plan will follow deliberate conclusions from team members.

Griffiths and Nugent (1998) list the final strategy as the celebration of success (i.e., the crisis prevention and response plan has ameliorated the particular challenging behavior). Although a positive outcome is desirable for the cohesiveness of the interdisciplinary team, challenging behaviors are often intractable and require the ongoing sustained attention from all members of the team.

The Team's Goal: Crisis Prevention

Although crisis response remains an important function of the interdisciplinary team, the ultimate goal is preventing challenging behavior from reaching crisis proportions. The interdisciplinary team is instrumental in designing a behavior support strategy minimizing the probability of a crisis situation. Crisis prevention requires a coordinated effort from the interdisciplinary team to develop an individualized plan for the client at risk. A number of steps are necessary for the development of a crisis prevention plan.

Identifying the Clients at Risk

The display of aberrant behavior patterns is evident to most care providers in their routine interactions with the client. However, many clients exhibit problem behaviors intermittently and in the presence of multiple setting events and antecedents. The frequency and severity of challenging behaviors become the primary consideration of whether an intervention plan needs to be developed for the client.

Identifying the Challenging Behaviors That May Result in Crisis

Severe aggressive and destructive behaviors, especially when the occurrence puts others in physical jeopardy, require a crisis prevention plan. Other behaviors, although not inherently aberrant, may require a crisis prevention plan. For example, removing one's clothing is not inherently aberrant, but if this behavior is performed in public, it becomes problematic. Likewise, leaving a work or residential site may be an appropriate behavior, but doing so without authorization or demonstrated safety skills may subject the individual to dangerous situations requiring crisis prevention planning.

Identifying the Variables Associated With Past Challenging Behavior

Once the client and the behaviors of concern have been recognized, it is essential to determine the functional variables that set the occasion for the display of challenging behavior. Especially critical in this process is identifying those setting events that serve as "establishing operations" affecting the occurrence of problem behaviors (Michael, 1982; Miltenberger, 1999). A number of methods for completing a functional assessment have been developed that identify the establishing operations, antecedent variables, and reinforcing consequences of problem behaviors. These are conducting an interview (e.g., Horner, Albin, Sprague, & Todd, 1999; O'Neill et al., 1997) or completing a rating scale (e.g., Durand, 1988; Durand & Crimmins, 1988; Iwata & DeLeon, 1995; March & Horner, 1998). The second method is used for direct observation of the client while engaging in the challenging behavior (e.g., Carr et al., 1994; O'Neill et al., 1997). The third method is through conducting a functional analysis by creating analog situations and noting the frequency of the target behavior under different environmental conditions (e.g., Iwata, Dorsey, Slifer, Bauman, & Richman, 1982; Miltenberger, 1999; O'Neill et al., 1997). Information obtained by an interview or rating scale must be buttressed by direct observation. Because methods of conducting a functional assessment vary in their usefulness and time expenditure, it is important that a designated individual of the interdisciplinary team be adept in conducting this assessment designed to define the patterns of challenging behavior, predict the occurrence and nonoccurrence, and identify the consequences maintaining the behavior (Horner et al., 1999).

Identifying Ecological Variables Associated With Challenging Behavior

The physical and social environments in which the client lives exert a major influence on behavior. It is important for the physical environment to promote appropriate behavior, not challenging behavior (Favell & McGimsey, 1993). To prevent a behavioral crisis, it is critical that the interdisciplinary team specifies what proximal and distal environmental features influence the occurrence of target behaviors that may escalate to crisis proportions.

Identifying the Skill Deficits That Make the Client Vulnerable to Challenging Behavior

The absence of appropriate skills in obtaining reinforcers from others may often result in challenging behavior. That is, the aberrant behavior may be reinforcing to both the client and the staff. Challenging behavior may be effective for the client in obtaining attention or escaping from nonpreferred settings or activities. Alternatively, by honoring the function of the client's aberrant behavior, staff can reduce the severity of challenging behavior. For example, a client may display self-injury and aggression to others to obtain staff attention. If staff members react to these behaviors, the problem behaviors are reinforced. Alternatively, staff's response of giving the client attention may be effective in curtailing self-injury and aggression. If effective in reducing challenging behaviors, attention is negatively reinforcing to staff members who are responding to the problem behaviors. Therefore, both the client's problem behavior and the staff response to it are reciprocally reinforced. These immediate reinforcing results have untoward lasting effects by strengthening the behaviors of concern. For crisis intervention, an inventory must be identified of skill deficits as well as skills in the client's repertoire that are not functional in obtaining reinforcers. The balance in efficiency of appropriate behavior versus challenging behavior in obtaining reinforcers becomes paramount. Efficiency is defined as (a) amount of physical effort, (b) the latency between the behavior and the reinforcer, and (c) the ratio of emitting the behavior and the reinforcing consequence. It is important for the client to acquire skills that are as efficient and effective as the challenging behavior in acquiring or removing desirable or undesirable events (cf. Horner & Day, 1991).

Identifying the Environmental Changes Important to Prevent Challenging Behavior

The research synthesis of positive behavior support (Carr et al., 1999) identified environmental changes from the research literature that were effective. Four factors were identified:

1. Interspersal training is the process by which a nonpreferred task is embedded within the context of preferred tasks, thus minimizing the occurrence of problem behaviors.

2. Providing an expansion of choices for the client in activities, tasks, and events. Increasing choices often correlates with a reduction in challenging behaviors.

3. Changing features that frequently evoke problem behaviors is often effective in reducing problem behaviors. For example, modifications in the duration of the task, the frequency of reinforcers during the task, and the clarity of behaviors needed to complete the task are often helpful in reducing problem behaviors.

4. Altering setting events is an environmental change that may have a positive effect in crisis prevention. Some examples of setting events influencing the occurrence of challenging behaviors include psychotropic medications, the presence of preferred caregivers, an environment containing pleasurable activities, and a comfortable sequencing of events.

These four environmental alterations in the physical, social, and procedural features are important for the interdisciplinary team to consider when planning for crisis prevention. The interdisciplinary team might also consider the common broad-based environmental changes such as a change from sheltered work to supported employment, adjustments in the structure of the physical environment to better accommodate the client's physical needs, modifications in the schedule of activities attuned to the client's preferences, and the enhancement of community-based activities providing more pleasant recreational pursuits and the opportunity to develop or foster friendships with others.

Identifying the Alternative Skills Needed to Control Challenging Behavior

An intervention strategy should include acquisition of appropriate skills that are functionally equivalent with challenging behavior in acquiring reinforcers (Carr, 1988). As previously mentioned, the trained alternative behavior must be at least as efficient and effective as the problem behavior in obtaining reinforcers. If not, then the alternative skill will not likely be demonstrated by the client. Three strategies from the research synthesis on positive behavior support pertain to the development of alternative skills (Carr et al., 1999):

1. Functional communication training. This training involves replacing the challenging behavior with a socially acceptable communicative behavior having identical functional properties. Functional communication may be accomplished verbally or, with nonverbal clients, gesturally. It is important that the desired communicative response effectively and efficiently competes with the challenging behavior. Continuously reinforcing the functional communication and not responding to the challenging behavior facilitates the efficiency of this desired behavior.

2. Self-management. This strategy teaches the client to control challenging behavior by self-imposed monitoring of behavior, evaluating the behavior of concern, and the delivering of consequences. As described by Gardner (1998b), teaching self-management to clients with intellectual disabilities is an important skill, especially because too frequently behavior is impulsively emitted through external provocation. This skill is helpful in reducing challenging behaviors and improving the client's independence.

3. Differential reinforcement of alternative behavior (DRA). This strategy encompasses both differential reinforcement of the desired behavior and planned ignoring of the challenging behavior. DRA generally refers to the topographical incompatibility of the desired and challenging behavior. Through differential reinforcement and planned ignoring, the frequency of desired behaviors increases while the frequency of challenging behaviors decreases.

Many practitioners and service providers have found that the following strategies have helped develop additional effective alternative skills: anger management, relaxation training, and social-skills training.

1. Anger management. This strategy is closely tied to self-management in that it teaches the client self-control skills to respond to anger-provoking situations in a socially appropriate manner (Benson, 1986; Novaco, 1975). Clients are taught to change their behavior in situations that are anger provoking by using problem-solving techniques rather than becoming assaultive or destructive. Anger management is frequently used in conjunction with other instructional programs.

2. Relaxation training. Training in this skill frequently offers an effective alternative to the display of challenging behavior (Bernstein & Borkovec, 1973; Cautela & Groden, 1978). The standard tension-release method involving 12 muscle groups and the frequency of training can be attuned to the client's need. Skill in this technique can be very helpful as an adjunct to anger management, as relaxation is a socially appropriate response to anger-provoking situations.

3. Improvement in social skills. Social skills training can be an effective strategy in teaching a client alternative response to challenging behaviors (King, Marcattilio, & Hanson, 1981; Liberman, DeRisi, & Mueser, 1989). By using a variety of behavioral methods (e.g., shaping, fading, differential reinforcement), this skill can be taught to clients in an individual or group format. These methods are helpful in teaching assertive skills for handling difficult situations.

Developing a Behavior Support Plan of Crisis Prevention

The development of a behavior support plan for crisis prevention requires the coordinated effort of members of an interdisciplinary team. This goal of preventing crises must be the driving force for effective results. Many techniques used in the development of an effective behavior support plan require the expertise of disciplines not usually available within the interdisciplinary team. Consequently, it is imperative to obtain consultants with the expertise needed to develop adequate crisis prevention and response.

Each of these steps is important for an effective interdisciplinary team. The next section will focus on the consultant's role as an important adjunctive staff person to the interdisciplinary team.

Consultant's Role in the Interdisciplinary Team

As stated above, a necessary component for crisis planning is the consultants who are active participants in the development of behavioral support plans for crisis prevention and response. Their suggestions must be congruent with the people and the environments where implementation will occur; that is, crisis plans presented to the interdisciplinary team need to be technically sound, but also compatible with the care providers' values and other factors associated with the client's care.

This congruence has been termed the *contextual* fit defined as "the congruence or compatibility that exists between specific features and components of a behavioral support plan and a variety of relevant variables relating to individuals and environments" (Albin, Lucyshyn, Horner, & Flannery, 1996, p. 82). The personal variables of the client, the values of the care providers conducting the support plan, and the environmental variables where the plan will be implemented are factors that must be considered. The consultant's challenge is to design a behavioral support plan grounded in the principles of behavior analysis that matches the values and resources of interdisciplinary team members. Otherwise, a technically sound behavioral support plan for crisis prevention and response may be developed, but it is unlikely it will succeed if the contextual match between the plan and the interdisciplinary team members implementing the plan is not achieved.

For the plan to be technically sound, it must be logically linked to the functional assessment conducted prior to the development of the behavioral support plan. Members of the interdisciplinary team need a consensus concerning the specific functions of the problem behavior in identified environments. For example, it is not sufficient to have merely a consensus that a problem behavior is escape motivated. The conditions under which the behavior occurs with an escape-motivated function need to be identified by the interdisciplinary team and incorporated in the behavioral support plan. The problem behavior may be escape motivated in performing nonpreferred cleaning tasks and transitional periods, but the acquisition of staff attention may be the function during community recreational activities. This requires a systematic review, situation by situation, throughout the day both at the day program and residence.

Although the behavioral support plan for crisis prevention and response is tailored for the individual at risk, it is important for interdisciplinary team members to recognize that the plan is developed for caregivers' behavior. It is unlikely a support plan will be implemented with fidelity if it is not congruent with implementors' level of skill, style of interaction shaped by values, and goals shared by the interdisciplinary team members.

Close contextual fit requires that support plan strategies are embedded in the client's normal rhythm of life: maintaining typical routines; the client's associations with others; and the activities in home, school, work, or events in the community — these are continued whenever possible unless it is evident that any of these significant variables put the client at risk of displaying challenging behaviors.

Once the behavioral support plan is developed and implemented, contextual fit must be maintained. This requires the consultant to have frequent interactions with members of the interdisciplinary team to obtain information about the workability of the support plan and comfort of caregivers in conducting the program. This interaction allows for fine tuning of critical components to maintain behavioral support. When members of the interdisciplinary team are involved in the functional assessment and behavioral support plan development, contextual fit is facilitated and occurs almost naturally.

The Interdisciplinary Team Meeting

The interdisciplinary team meeting is the cornerstone when building crisis prevention and response plans. It involves a three-phase process: (a) premeeting planning, (b) the meeting process, (c) action following the meeting (Delaney & Clausen, 1997). Each phase will be described to ensure that meetings, especially those pertaining to crisis prevention and response, are effective in achieving their stated purpose.

Premeeting Planning

The first step is an invitation by the coordinator to the members of the interdisciplinary team stating the date, time, location, and purpose of the meeting. The next item is having the agenda distributed prior to the meeting. The agenda consists of a title referring to the purpose of the meeting, the date and location of the meeting, and the topics according to preestablished time lines (see Figure 13.1).

The top of the agenda lists the four key roles for different interdisciplinary team members during the meeting. The first is the facilitator. This team member is responsible for leading the discussion on the agenda and ensuring the team remains task oriented. The second is the recorder. This individual takes notes of the discussion and issues during the meeting. The third is the time keeper. This person prompts the interdisciplinary team members to limit unnecessary discussion and follow the agenda time lines. The fourth key role is the process observer. This individual's role is to ensure that team members are interacting respectfully and that all opinions and observations are acknowledged. If interruptions or side conversations occur, the process observer helps refocus the team.

The body of the agenda is divided into four columns. The time frames are in the left-hand column; the second column consists of the topic of discussion within the time frame; the third is the person responsible for leading the discussion or reporting information germane to the discussion; and the last column presents a brief description of the topic area or issue to be discussed. Having a block of time dedicated to additional discussion, which was not adequately covered during the time constraints of the agenda, is frequently useful. This time block also prompts interdisciplinary team members to limit discussion relevant to

---

Interdisciplinary Team Meeting

Date:

Roles: Facilitator:
       Recorder:
       Time Keeper:
       Process Observer:

Time:	Issue:	By Whom:	Comment:
9:00–9:10	Review of last minutes and items added to the agenda	Everyone	Changes to be recorded in current minutes and adjust agenda
9:10–9:40			
9:40–9:55			
9:55–10:00			
10:00–10:15	Break	Everyone	
10:15–10:30			
10:30–10:45			
10:45–10:55	Around the horn	Everyone	Ask each member if there is any comment he or she wishes to offer (e.g., new activities, upcoming events, interesting professional reading, etc.)
10:55–11:00	Process observer's report Roles for next meeting Date of next meeting:	Facilitator: Recorder: Time Keeper: Process Observer:	

Figure 13.1. Interdisciplinary team meeting sample agenda. The time allotment, issues discussed, and the comments vary in each meeting.

the agenda with knowledge that additional pertinent issues can be discussed during this time.

The Meeting Process

The facilitator is responsible for following the meeting agenda. Prior to the agenda items, the facilitator should introduce all team members and give their relationship with the client. The first item on the agenda is the review of the previous meeting minutes and the opportunity for additional items to be added to the agenda. The facilitator briefly introduces each item on the agenda; the recorder, time keeper, and process observer fulfill their assigned tasks. It is important that resolution be achieved on each agenda item. Because this meeting, as described, pertains to crisis prevention and response for a focus client, a simple decision that a positive behavioral support plan will be created will not be adequate. The lead person will need to be identified in the creation of the support plan for crisis prevention and the manner by which the person obtains a contextual fit will be described. The date by which the positive behavioral support plan will be established and the in-services also described. This may or may not call for a follow-up interdisciplinary team meeting to ensure achievement of the goals of providing behavioral support.

Action Subsequent to the Meeting

The recorder who wrote the meeting minutes distributes them to all interdisciplinary team members. Distributing the minutes to team members who did not attend the meeting is especially important. The minutes list the meeting date, location, purpose, and individuals present. The body of the minutes consists of four categories in a format similar to Figure 13.1: Problem-Issue, Solution-Task, Who (i.e., the person responsible), By When (i.e., the date when the solution or task will be resolved). Usually many tasks are assigned during the interdisciplinary team meeting and subsequent meetings should be scheduled. For example, if a positive behavioral support plan draft is developed, the specialist will want to ensure that a contextual fit exists with all members of the interdisciplinary team. In addition, the interdisciplinary team meeting is an ideal time to (a) schedule a functional assessment interview, (b) examine what environmental modification can be made to reduce the likelihood of crisis response, and (c) in-service staff on the support plan components for both crisis prevention and response. Consequently, more than one client's support plan may be on the agenda for any given meeting. Typically, frequent follow-up interdisciplinary team meetings or meetings with key caregivers of the team are made in the initial stages of the plan. Once the plan is developed, frequent follow-up evaluations need to be scheduled and completed to ensure that (a) crisis situations are eliminated or reduced to a near zero level and (b) the environment is structured so that the person receives activity patterns, social networks, a level of independence, and access to preferred events to produce a quality of life valued and enjoyed by the individual.

Summary

This chapter presented the essential components of, the primary goal of, the role of consultants in, and the meeting process of an interdisciplinary team targeting crisis prevention and response. For the interdisciplinary team to be optimally effective, each member must have a common goal of preventing crisis situations vis-à-vis responding with interdisciplinary team involvement only when crisis response is necessary. The opinions of each member, regardless of his or her interaction with the focus client, must be valued and considered when planning for crisis prevention. Having an effective behavior support plan designed with the input from all interdisciplinary team members frequently results in clients living in least-restrictive environments, enjoying a quality life, and being integrated in community-based vocational and recreational activities.

References

Albin, R. W., Lucyshyn, J. M., Horner, R. H., & Flannery, K. B. (1996). Contextual fit for behavioral support plans: A model for "Goodness of Fit." In L. K. Koegel, R. L. Koegel, & G. Dunlap (Eds.), *Positive behavioral support: Including people with difficult behavior in the community* (pp. 81–98). Baltimore: Paul H. Brookes.

American Psychiatric Association. (1994). *Diagnostic and statistical manual of mental disorders* (4th ed.). Washington, DC: Author.

Benson, B. A. (1986). Anger management training. *Psychiatric Aspects of Mental Retardation Reviews, 5,* 51–55.

Berstein, D. A., & Borkovec, T. D. (1973). *Progressive relaxation training: A manual for the helping professions.* Champaign, IL: Research Press.

Carr, E. G. (1988). Functional equivalence as a mechanism of response generalization. In R. H. Horner, G. Dunlap, & R. L. Koegel (Eds.), *Generalization and maintenance: Life-style changes in applied settings* (pp. 221–241). Baltimore: Paul H. Brookes.

Carr, E. G., Horner, R. H., Turnbull, A. P., Marquis, J. G., McLaughlin, D. M., McAtee, M. L., Smith, C. E, Ryan, K. A., Ruef, M. B., & Doolabh, A. (1999). *Positive behavior support for people with developmental disabilities: A research synthesis.* Washington, DC: American Association on Mental Retardation.

Carr, E. G., Levin, L., McConnachie, G., Carlson, J. I, Kemp, D. C., & Smith, C. E. (1994). *Communication-based intervention for problem behavior: A user's guide for producing positive change.* Baltimore: Paul H. Brookes.

Cautela, J. R., & Groden, J. (1978). *Relaxation: A comprehensive manual for adults, children, and children with special needs.* Champaign, IL: Research Press.

Delaney, M. J., & Clausen, B. J. (1997). *Beyond the storm into synergy.* Unpublished manuscript.

Doss, L. S., & Reichle, J. (1991). Replacing excess behavior with an initial communicative repertoire. In J. Reichle, J. York, & J. Sigafoos (Eds.), *Implementing augmentative and alternative communication: Strategies for learners with severe disabilities* (pp. 215–237). Baltimore: Paul H. Brookes.

Durand, V. M. (1988). The motivation assessment scale. In M. Hersen & A. S. Bellack (Eds.), *Dictionary of behavioral assessment techniques.* New York: Pergamon Press.

Durand, V. M., & Crimmins, D. B. (1988). *The motivation assessment scale: An administration manual.* Unpublished manuscript. Albany: State University of New York at Albany.

Favell, J. E., & McGimsey, J. F. (1993). Defining an acceptable treatment environment. In R. Van Houten & S. Axelrod (Eds.), *Behavior analysis and treatment* (pp. 25–45). New York: Plenum Press.

Gardner, W. I. (1998a). Initiating the case formulation process. In D. M. Griffith, W. I. Gardner, & J. Nugent (Eds.), *Individual centered behavioral interventions: A multimodal functional approach* (pp. 17–65). Kingston, NY: NADD Press.

Gardner, W. I. (1998b). Teaching skills of self-management In D. M. Griffith, W. I. Gardner, & J. Nugent (Eds.), *Individual centered behavioral interventions: A multimodal functional approach* (pp. 259–273). Kingston, NY: NADD Press.

Gates, J. R. (1999). Adverse behavioral effects of antiepileptic medications in people with developmental disabilities. In N. A. Wieseler & R. H. Hanson (Eds.), *Challenging behavior of persons with mental health disorders and severe developmental disabilities* (pp. 113–123). Washington, DC: American Association on Mental Retardation.

Griffiths, D. M., & Nugent, J. A. (1998). Creating an integrated service system. In D. M. Griffith, W. I. Gardner, & J. A. Nugent (Eds.), *Individual centered behavioral interventions: A multimodal functional approach* (pp. 219–238). Kingston, NY: NADD Press.

Grossman, H. J. (Ed.). (1983). *Classification in mental retardation.* Washington, DC: American Association on Mental Deficiency.

Horner, R. H., Albin, R. W., Sprague, J. R., & Todd, A. W. (1999). Positive behavior support. In M. E. Snell & F. Brown (Eds.), *Instruction of students with severe disabilities* (5th ed.) (pp. 207–244). Upper Saddle River, NJ: Prentice Hall.

Horner, R. H., & Day, H. M. (1991). The effects of response efficiency on functionally equivalent competing behaviors. *Journal of Applied Behavior Analysis, 24,* 265–278.

Iwata, B. A., & DeLeon, I. G. (1995). *The functional analysis screening tool (FAST).* Unpublished manuscript, University of Florida, Gainesville.

Iwata, B. A., Dorsey, M. F., Slifer, K. J., Bauman, K. E., & Richman, G. S. (1982). *Analysis and Intervention in Developmental Disabilities, 2,* 3–20.

Kern, C. A. (1999). Psychopharmacotherapy for people with profound and severe mental retardation and mental disorders. In N. A. Wieseler & R. H. Hanson (Eds.), *Challenging behavior of persons with mental health disorders and severe developmental disabilities* (pp.103–112). Washington, DC: American Association on Mental Retardation.

Kincaid, D. (1996). Person-centered planning. In L. K. Koegel, R. L. Koegel, & G. Dunlap (Eds.), *Positive behavioral support: Including people with difficult behavior in the community* (pp. 439–465). Baltimore: Paul H. Brookes.

King, R. P., Marcattilio, A. J. M., & Hanson, R. H. (1981). Some functions of videotape equipment in training social skills in institutionalized developmentally retarded adults. *Behavioral Engineering, 6*(4), 159–167.

Liberman, R. P., DeRisi, W. J., & Mueser, K. T. (1989). *Social skills training for psychiatric patients.* New York: Pergamon Press.

Luckasson, R., Coulter, D. L., Polloway, E. A., Reiss, S., Schalock, R. L., Snell, M. E., Spitalnik, D. M., & Stark, J. A. (1992). *Mental retardation: Diagnosis, classification, and systems of support* (9th ed.). Washington, DC: American Association on Mental Retardation.

March, R., & Horner, R. (1998, May). *School-wide behavioral support: Extending the impact of ABA by expanding the unit of analysis.* Presentation at the Association for Behavior Analysis annual convention, Orlando, FL.

Michael, J. (1982). Distinguishing between discriminative and motivational functions of stimuli. *Journal of the Experimental Analysis of Behavior, 37,* 149–155.

Miltenberger, R. G. (1999). Understanding problem behaviors through functional assessment. In N. A. Wieseler & R. H. Hanson (Eds.), *Challenging behavior of persons with mental health disorders and severe developmental disabilities* (pp. 215–235). Washington, DC: American Association on Mental Retardation.

Novaco, R. W. (1975). *Anger control: The development and evaluation of an experimental treatment.* Lexington, MA: Heath.

O'Neill, R. E., Horner, R. H., Albin, R. W., Sprague, J. R., Storey, K., & Newton, J. S. (1997). *Functional assessment and program development for problem behavior: A practical handbook.* Cincinnati: Brooks/Cole.

Rainforth, B., & York-Barr, J. (1997). Strategies for implementing collaborative teamwork. In B. Rainforth & J. York-Barr (Eds.), *Collaborative teams for students with severe disabilities: Integrating therapy and educational services* (2nd ed., pp. 247–303). Baltimore: Paul H. Brookes.

Discussion

Ronald H. Hanson
Mount Olivet Rolling Acres
Victoria, Minnesota

Norman A. Wieseler
Eastern Minnesota Community Support Services
Faribault, Minnesota

Prompted by the reduction and eventual closing of institutions, crisis prevention and response have emerged as a key necessity in supporting the community placements of individuals leaving the institutions and those with developmental disabilities who lived with their families or in other community-based arrangements. Many locales have reported that clients with histories of serious challenging behaviors are also likely to have concurrent mental health disorders. This monograph addresses the groundwork for developing crisis services, details useful treatment options, describes the manner in which interventions are delivered, and presents specialized treatment options beneficial for many clients receiving crisis prevention and response services.

Generally, as the public becomes aware of the availability of specialized crisis services, the need expands. Many clients never receive attention from governmental or private agencies until their providers become aware of the availability of specialized services.

Varieties and dissimilarities of the manner in which services are delivered indicate that crisis prevention and response services do not conform to a nationwide set of standards. As this monograph shows, treatment needs and resources differ among states. The cited experiences from a variety of locations, especially where deinstitutionalization has rapidly proceeded, suggest effective options in providing crisis prevention and response.

One common element noted in this volume was the level of expertise in providing crisis services. Expertise in positive behavioral support and the creation of intervention plans within the context of an effective interdisciplinary team was essential for preventing and responding to challenging behavior. When mental health disorders are coupled with challenging behavior, professionals in psychiatric disciplines also become necessary.

As several authors in this text advocate, the most effective crisis prevention and response services should occur where the client lives, works, or goes to school. Just seeing a counselor in an office will likely be insufficient as an intervention. In planning for crisis services, some combination of outreach and residential care is often necessary. This monograph highlights many differing services tailored to the recipient's needs. Some clients can be served where they live and work. Others may need services in a different location such as a temporary crisis home, specialized service residence, or setting affiliated with a university.

The development of crisis prevention and response is usually well received by county social workers, residential and day program staff, families, and other care providers. When the development of crisis services is proposed as revenue neutral or saving taxpayers' money, it usually has been supported by legislators. What is generally spent on psychiatric hospitalization can be spent more wisely on crisis prevention and response, which can greatly reduce most psychiatric hospitalizations for individuals with developmental disabilities. In a managed care environment, psychiatric hospitals have also generally appreciated the development of community-based outpatient crisis services. Advocacy groups have been strong supporters of alternative community-based crisis prevention and support.

It is anticipated that many states without crisis prevention and response services will develop them in the future. As institutions downsize and close, the need for crisis services becomes paramount. The high cost associated with the lack of development for alternative community support services must be recognized as institutions reduce in size and eventually close. Ongoing treatment requires the commitment of service providers using valid and accepted principles of behavior support. This monograph provides helpful suggestions for states serving only a subgroup of clients needing specialized care. It also provides a useful guidepost for states developing crisis xs in the future.